D0090471

JANUARY
FIRST

JANUARY FIRST

A Child's Descent into Madness and Her
Father's Struggle to Save Her

MICHAEL SCHOFIELD

CROWN PUBLISHERS
NEW YORK

Published in the United States by Crown Publishers,
an imprint of the Crown Publishing Group,
a division of Random House, Inc., New York.
www.crownpublishing.com

CROWN and the Crown colophon are registered trademarks
of Random House, Inc.

Permission to reproduce lyrics to "Yellow Submarine" provided by © 1966
Sony-ATV Music Publishing LLC. All rights administered by Sony-ATV
Music Publishing LLC, 8 Music Square West, Nashville, TN 37203.
All rights reserved. Used by permission.

Library of Congress Cataloging-in-Publication Data
Schofield, Michael, 1976–
January first: a child's descent into madness and her father's struggle
to save her / Michael Schofield.—1st ed.
1. Schofield, January, 2002– 2. Schizophrenia in children—Patients—
Biography. 3. Schizophrenics—Family relationships. I. Title.
RJ506.S3S36 2011
618.92'8980092—dc23
[B] 2011049462

ISBN 978-0-307-71908-9
eISBN 978-0-307-71910-2

Printed in the United States of America

Book design by Maria Elias
Jacket design by Laura Duffy
Jacket photograph by James Walker / Trevillion Images

10 9 8 7 6 5 4 3 2 1

First Edition

For Jani, Bodhi, Susan, and Honey . . .
Thank you for your patience and your faith. I love you.

AUTHOR'S NOTE

While this is a true story, certain names and details have been changed to protect the identities of those who appear within.

FOREWORD

Schizophrenia is a little like cancer. You can't trust that it will ever go away completely. Even if one is asymptomatic, once cancer has been inside your body, the chances of it coming back remain forever until the day you die. Years of trial and error have given my daughter a combination of medications that keep the worst of her schizophrenic symptoms under control. The hallucinations are still present, but now it's more like having a TV show on in the background with the volume turned down. Most of the time it doesn't interrupt her functioning in our world. But there are other times when the volume rises and becomes so demanding of her attention that she is lost within that world, unable to differentiate between reality and fantasy.

Four years ago, I was convinced that schizophrenia would take my daughter completely. But by the efforts of everyone in her life, we turned the tide back. We stopped its advance across her mind and turned the volume back down.

Nobody knows what causes schizophrenia. Studies are rare. The prevailing theory right now is that it is a bio-chemical defect in the brain (generally referred to as the "Biological Model of Mental Illness"), possibly a degenerative neural disorder closer to Alzheimer's.

In dealing with it, sometimes I feel as if I'm carrying a flashlight around inside a dark tunnel, stumbling, trying to feel my way as I go, praying the batteries won't die until I can reach the light at the end of the tunnel. Needless to say, I've tripped along the way. Yes, there are plenty of things I regret, moments with Jani I wish I would have handled differently if I could do it over again. Unfortunately, I can't go back in time. I can't change what happened in the past. All I can do is move forward and keep trying to be the father Jani needs me to be.

This book should not be taken as a ringing endorsement of what to do when your child goes to a place you can't understand. Rather, it's simply my family's story of trying to find our way out of the dark.

During one stay in the hospital, while my wife, Susan, and I were visiting our daughter, Jani looked down from her fourth-floor window and said, "I want to jump down."

I was busy trying to keep our son, Bodhi, engaged with the video game we were playing on a hospital computer. I heard her clearly, but I do what I usually do when I hear things like that: try to distract her.

"You don't want to do that," I replied, as calmly as I could. "Come here and play with me and Bodhi."

Out of the corner of my eye, I could see she was still looking down.

"I want to die," she said softly.

I stiffened. It had been a long time since I'd heard her say anything like that. "I thought you wanted to live to one hundred," I chuckled nervously.

"I want to die at nine."

I reached out for her. "Why? Why do you want to die?"

She turned to look at me. "Because I have schizophrenia."

There was nothing psychotic about her statement. It was actually quite lucid. Jani was simply sad. Susan and I were not sure what to do.

I immediately left a message for the doctor, who checked with her the next day. She repeated the same thing to him. He asked her what she believed it means to have schizophrenia.

"I see and hear stuff that isn't there," she told him.

MY FIRST WRITING about Jani was on my Facebook page. I wrote to vent, but soon realized that I was also trying to make sense of what was happening to my daughter and my family. My Facebook posts evolved into a blog, and I started writing more. When our story became public, hundreds of families emailed me, all telling a variation of the same message: "We thought we were alone." Encouraged by the inspiration I'd gotten and hoping to help other families dealing with similar problems, I formed a private online support group where parents could talk to one another without fear of criticism, primarily from the anti-psychiatry movement, which, though it has many faces, basically denies that mental illness exists. They certainly cannot accept that it happens in children. Nevertheless, from my blog posts they drew conclusions, based on what they believe, that I abused my daughter and that the true cause of Jani's condition rests in her parents and how she was raised.

I struggled for years to understand how, in the early twenty-first century, some people, even doctors, could be so unwilling to believe in child-onset schizophrenia. I'm still amazed at how many people write to me saying Jani is possessed by demons that must be exorcised. Really, it's all the same thing: denial.

But when Jani said to me that she wanted to die, I finally understood where that denial comes from. Some people hang on to the abuse assumption or the demon theory because those things can be controlled. The idea that there is a disease out there that is totally arbitrary is terrifying. If Jani can develop schizophrenia, any of us can. And the idea that all it might take is the crossing of some wires in the brain is more than some people can handle.

I understand. Nobody wants a child to suffer, so we come up with any explanation we can for why it is happening.

But denial is not going to help Jani or any of the other mentally ill and schizophrenic children I have come to know. What they need is acceptance. What they need is for us to be telling them "your illness does not define you."

We cannot go inside their minds and "fix" them. But we can fix the world so they can live in it.

Schizophrenia is not a death sentence. It is a disease that can and must be managed. But it is also just another part of the rich rainbow of humanity.

I want Jani to see that rainbow. And I want you to see it, too.

That is why I wrote this book.

This is not a requiem for a child. This is a journey out of darkness and into the light.

PROLOGUE

June 2006

M ost three-year-olds are in bed by now, but most three-year-olds are not geniuses like my daughter. She can read, calculate multiplication and division in her head, and even quiz my wife, Susan, and me on the periodic table using her place mat with all the elements on it.

It's almost 9 P.M., and Susan finishes her shift reporting news and traffic for a radio station in Los Angeles at 7 P.M. Allowing for traffic, she's probably just getting home right now, but still I wait. I want to keep Janni out until there is nowhere left to go but home. We've been doing this since Janni was an infant. At that time I would take her to IKEA, where we'd play in the ball pit and I'd throw balls at my head and she would laugh hysterically. When I'm lecturing at Cal State Northridge, it's Susan who's making the rounds with Janni, but tonight I'm on duty.

As I watch her, running ahead of me into the mall, the only place still open at this hour, I wonder how she keeps going. We've already been to the LA Zoo, IKEA, and a McDonald's play area—anything that will engage Janni's mind, even for a little while. We have season passes to the zoo, and her favorite part is when we go under a tunnel and then pop our heads up into the ground like prairie dogs. Janni loves dogs. She'll even call people "dogs," which I worry someone might take the wrong way.

She has to be well past the point of physical exhaustion by now, but if she is she doesn't show it. Not that it matters. It's not her body. It's her mind. I have to wear out her mind. That has been the only way to get her to sleep since she was born.

The mall is almost empty, which is a good thing. The fewer people the better.

Janni storms into a toy store, one of the high-end places that sell classic toys. The clerk comes over to us.

"Can I help you?" she asks.

"No, thanks. Just looking," I say, wanting to get rid of her as soon as possible. The last thing I want is for Janni to start talking to her. Janni doesn't talk like your average three-year-old.

The clerk nods and starts to walk away, but to my dismay Janni follows her.

"I have seven rats at home," Janni tells her.

"Wow," she replies, surprised. "You have seven rats?"

"Yep." Janni nods. "I call them Monday, Tuesday, Wednesday, Thursday, Friday, Saturday, and Sunday."

Then comes the part I hate the most. The clerk looks up at me, a questioning expression on her face. She is looking to me, the dad, for confirmation of this incredible fact. One rat she could understand, even two or three, but seven? Except that we don't have any rats. Every single one of them is an imaginary friend.

Janni's first imaginary friend, a dog named Low, appeared right before her third birthday. Then came a cat named 400. By now, I've lost count of how many she has. They all come from a place called Calilini, which Janni describes as a desert island off the coast of California.

Normally, this would be no big deal. Everybody knows that little kids have imaginations. But Janni gets so angry when I dismiss her friends like that. She looks at me like I've betrayed her.

I open my mouth, about to say, *Well, we don't really. They're actually imaginary rats,* but I see Janni turn to me, awaiting my response. Right now, she seems content. If I tell the clerk the truth, I know what will happen. Janni will emit one of her earsplitting screams. Then she'll grab things off the shelf and throw them on the floor. I will tell her to pick them up, because I really do try to reinforce good behavior. But then Janni will say, *No,* like a petulant teenager and run out of the store. I'll call, *Janni, you need to come back here and pick this stuff up!* but she'll be gone. Then I'll have to abandon the mess she made and chase her for fear of losing her. I will come out of the store and see her about a hundred feet down the mall, looking back at me, waiting.

It suddenly occurs to me . . . *Why do I have to tell the truth? This woman is never going to come over to our apartment. She will never know that we really don't have seven rats. Why make Janni feel more different than she already is?*

I nod and spread my hands in a *Yes . . . I know it's crazy* expression. "That's right. Seven rats."

She shakes her head.

"Wow." Her eyes widen, giving me a look like I'm nuts, but I don't care about that. I just want to keep the peace.

I come over to Janni.

"Okay, Janni, let's go." I rush her along to avoid digging a deeper hole for myself.

"Do you want to meet Friday?" Janni suddenly asks her.

Oh, shit, I think nervously.

"Come on, Janni. We have to go. We need to get home and feed our rats."

The clerk looks at Janni, confused.

"Do I want to meet Friday?" she repeats.

"She's one of my rats," Janni says earnestly, her face completely straight. "I have her right here in my pocket."

The clerk looks up at me in horror.

"You have a rat with you?! You can't bring animals into the store!" She moves toward the phone on the counter, ready to call security. *Dammit!*

"It's okay," Janni says, chasing after her. "She won't bite." She comes up behind the clerk and holds out her empty palm. "See? She's a nice rat."

The clerk stares at Janni's empty palm, the phone halfway to her ear, before she realizes what is happening.

Finally, she chuckles nervously. "Oh, my God," she says, looking over at me. "She had me going there for a minute. I thought you really had a rat with you."

"We do," Janni says, her face totally serious. "We brought Friday. Here she is." She extends her palm into the clerk's face, as if she's nearsighted.

"Janni, come on," I call, desperately wanting to leave.

The clerk smiles and pretends to pat the rat.

"He's a very nice rat," she tells Janni.

I wince. I can hear the condescension in her voice. She is treating Janni like every other child, believing Janni isn't smart enough to know she's being blown off.

"She," Janni corrects.

"She." The clerk nods, looking up at me with an expression I get all the time: *Your daughter has a wonderful imagination.* Then she smiles at Janni.

"Do you like to pretend?"

Janni doesn't answer. I see a look of frustatration come over her face. Suddenly, she grabs several classic wooden games off the shelf and throws them down on the floor.

"Janni, stop that!" I run over and grab her hands to stop her. She pulls free and runs deeper into the store, pulling items off the shelf and throwing them down.

I chase after her. "Janni!" But I know it doesn't matter what I say to Janni now. She won't stop. I will have to drag her out of the store. I'm angry at Janni, but even angrier at the stupid clerk. *Why couldn't she just play along?* I know it's unfair of me to expect the world to play along with Janni's imagination. But that doesn't stop me from wishing they would.

CHAPTER ONE

August 8, 2006

Today is Janni's fourth birthday, and I'm setting up her pool party at the clubhouse in our apartment complex.

I place pool toys in the water. Janni is already splashing around.

"Come in, Daddy!"

"I'm coming, Janni. I just have to finish setting up."

"Look, Janni!" Susan calls out. "Lynn and the twins are here. Come say hi."

I look over to the gate where Susan is letting them in. Janni is the same age as the twins. We've known them since they were babies.

"Janni?" Susan calls again to her. "Come say hi to Lynn and the twins."

"No," Janni calls back, not even bothering to turn around and see.

"Janni, you have to welcome your guests," Susan says, a bit more sternly.

"No!" Janni yells behind her, more forcefully this time.

"Hi, January!" Lynn calls. "Happy birthday!"

"I'm not January!" Janni screams, still not turning around. Then calmly, "I'm Blue-Eyed Tree Frog."

Lynn is visibly taken aback a little, but recovers quickly; she's known our struggle with Janni's constant name changing for a while now.

A year ago, Janni stopped going by her name. And this phase has gone on way longer than we thought it would. Whenever someone calls her by her real name, she screams like somebody put her hand to a hot frying pan.

We don't even try to force her to use her given name. At this point we're happy if she just picks one name and sticks with it. The problem is that she changes it all the time, sometimes multiple times in the same day. She's been "Hot Dog," "Rainbow," "Firefly," and now "Blue-Eyed Tree Frog," which was originally "Red-Eyed Tree Frog," from *Go Diego! Go!*, until a lady working at Sav-On drugstore pointed out, "But you have blue eyes, dear."

"Lynn and the girls have come to your birthday party," Susan reminds her. "You need to come and greet them."

Janni gets out of the pool and comes over to the twins. She is not pouting. She is smiling and rubbing her hands rapidly, as if she is actually suddenly happy to see them. It's like the previous outburst never happened.

Susan gets the twins two juice boxes from the cooler.

"Hi, Janni. How are you?" Lynn asks pleasantly.

The hand rubbing stops and the smile vanishes. "I'm not Janni! I'm Blue-Eyed Tree Frog."

"Oh, I'm sorry. I forgot." Lynn quickly corrects herself like she just received a mild electric shock.

"Girls, wish Blue-Eyed Tree Frog a happy birthday," Lynn instructs her daughters.

"Happy birthday, Janni," they dutifully intone. The twins have known my daughter as Janni since before they could talk. It is all they know.

"I'm not Janni!" she screams at the twins. "I'm Blue-Eyed Tree Frog."

The twins look up at their mom, confused.

"Janni!" Susan warns. "Be polite."

I say nothing. Sure, I would like Janni to be polite, but I realize odd behavior is a by-product of her genius. She hit all of her developmental markers early and was already talking at eight months. By thirteen months she knew all her letters, both big and small, even if they were turned on their side or upside down. Then, at eighteen months, she was speaking in grammatically correct sentences, introducing herself to people saying, "I'm Janni Paige and I am eighteen months old."

But I didn't fully comprehend what she was capable of until I came back from grad school one evening when Janni was two and Susan was telling me about their day.

"I've been teaching her addition," Susan told me, which I already knew, "so today we started on subtraction. I asked her what 'seven minus four' was."

"Did she get it right?" I asked.

"Yes, she did, so we did 'seven minus three is four.' Then she asks me, 'Mommy, what's four minus seven?' so I started trying to explain negative numbers to her."

I stare at Susan. "She asked you what was four minus seven?"

Susan, washing dishes, turns to me. "Yeah." She sees the look of shock on my face. "What's wrong?"

"She asked you that right out of the blue?"

"Yes. What is it?"

Negative numbers, I remember thinking. Negative numbers are a totally abstract concept because they don't exist in the real world. You can't see negative four apples. At two years old, Janni's mind made the jump from what Piaget called "concrete reasoning" to "abstract reasoning," something that typically happens at a much older age. Janni could conceive of concepts that did not actually physically exist.

I have fantasies of Janni going to Harvard or Yale or MIT before she is even a teenager. My ultimate dream, when I close my eyes at night, is Janni winning the Nobel Prize. For what, I don't know and don't really care. But to be able to do what she can do at two years old, she must be a gift to humanity. I think that trumps being impolite on occasion.

"Would you like some juice?" Susan hands the twins the juice boxes and they take them.

Janni starts to laugh and flings her arm at the twins. "400 is splashing mango juice on you," she chortles, without touching them.

The girls flinch instinctively, then look up at their mother for guidance, not sure what happened.

"400 is splashing mango juice on you." Janni makes the move again like she is throwing juice on the twins, but she has nothing in her hand.

The twins retreat to either side of their mother.

"Janni, that isn't nice," Susan corrects.

"But it's not me. It's 400. 400 is splashing mango juice on them. She likes to splash mango juice on people." Her arm shoots out with the imaginary juice again. We don't even have mango juice.

The twins look up at Lynn. "You both need sunscreen." She looks down at them, taking each daughter in one hand and over to the lounge chairs and tables.

"Well then, tell 400 to stop," Susan tells Janni. "400 is another one of her imaginary friends," she explains to Lynn.

Janni turns away and says to the air, "400, stop that." She waits, apparently for a response, before turning back to the twins.

"She won't stop." Janni breaks into laughter again. "It is so funny. 400 is throwing mango juice on you."

The twins are clearly scared, as Lynn puts on their sunscreen. "It's okay, we know Janni is 'unique.'"

This is frustrating. She's being imaginative, but the twins haven't seen imagination like this. Geniuses are often eccentric, I think to myself.

"Janni!" Susan's voice goes up an octave. "Stop it!"

"It's not me! It's 400!"

"You control 400. Tell her to stop."

Janni puts out her hands in exasperation. "I can't!"

"Janni . . . ," Susan begins, but I cut her off.

"Let it go."

Janni comes over to me and and we get ready to go into the pool. This is what I do. I am her protector from the rest of the world.

I see the look of frustration on Susan's face, but she doesn't completely understand Janni like I do.

"She needs to greet her friends," she tells me imploringly. "You're not helping her learn to be polite."

"It's her birthday. Let it go," I reply.

Susan opens her mouth to protest.

"Let it go," I say again, more firmly. Susan closes her mouth and gives me an annoyed look.

I jump in the water and come up to the edge, holding out my arms. "Come on, Janni. Jump to me."

"400 wants to jump in, too," Janni says earnestly.

"Cats don't generally like water."

"Okay, you stay here, 400."

Janni jumps to me, and I carry her out into the middle of the pool. Janni suddenly looks back at the edge.

"Oh, no! 400 fell in the pool!" she cries out. "400, don't drown!"

"I got 400," I answer. I put Janni down in the shallow end and wade over to where I imagine 400 to be. This is what I do that makes me different from everybody else in Janni's life. I play along with her imaginary friends like they are real. I'll be damned if I'm going to get lumped in with the "thirteens" in her mind. Janni says "thirteens" are kids and adults who don't have her imagination. She considers herself a "twenty," like me, and Susan a "seventeen," while most of her friends are "fifteens." But the "thirteens" have no imagination at all.

"Got her!" I fish nothing out of the water. "Ah! Now she is on my head! 400!" I pretend to sink under the weight of the imaginary cat. I will not shut any aspect of Janni down. I will not restrict anything, because I worry once she shuts down in order to conform, her full potential might be lost.

Janni smiles and laughs.

"400! Get off Daddy's head."

I smile back, happy.

"You know, Janni, if you could find an ocean big enough to put Saturn in it, it would float." This is how I teach her. I engage her imaginary friends and then she pays attention.

"Do you remember what the atmospheric pressure on Venus is?"

"Ninety," Janni answers.

"That's right. You would weigh ninety times what you weigh on Earth. Of course, if we were on Venus right now, we'd be swimming in sulfuric acid. And then there is the heat. Venus is hotter than Mercury, even though Mercury is closer to the sun, about eight hundred degrees Fahrenheit."

"It gets up to two hundred degrees in Calilini," Janni says.

Here is my chance to insert a little reality into her world.

"Janni, that's hotter than any place on Earth. That's nearly the boiling point of water. Nothing could survive that temperature."

"My friends do."

"It's not possible. Our bodies are mostly made of water, and at that temperature we would literally start to boil. How can they possibly survive?"

Janni shrugs. "They do."

I open my mouth, ready to continue arguing the illogic of this, but Janni is drifting away from me so I let it drop.

"Janni," I call.

She turns around.

"I still have a cat on my head."

She smiles.

I AM LOOKING at the pizza boxes on the table.

Last year, I ordered six medium cheese pizzas and we ran out before all the guests had even arrived, so Susan wanted me to order nine this time. I did, except that now six of them sit still unopened.

Susan comes over and tells me it is time to do the cake.

"Have you told everybody to sing 'Happy Birthday' to Blue-Eyed Tree Frog?" I ask her.

"Yes, I have," Susan replies, knowing my fear and hers. The last thing we both want is Janni flipping out on her birthday. "Hopefully, people will remember." She turns and calls out that it is time to light the candles.

Everybody gathers around the cake, which even says, HAPPY BIRTHDAY, BLUE-EYED TREE FROG.

"Okay, you ready?" Susan asks me.

I light the candles. Janni stands between us, rubbing her hands at a speed so fast it looks like it must be painful on her wrists, but she shows no discomfort.

"Okay . . . ," Susan begins. "Happy birthday to you . . ."

Everybody sings along. "Happy birthday to you. Happy birthday, dear . . ."

Susan looks at me, nervously.

I sing ". . . Blue Eyed Tree Frog" at the top of my lungs, trying to lead the guests in the correct name and cut off any "mistakes" before Janni can hear them.

"Happy birthday to you!"

Everybody claps, including Janni. I look up at Susan and see her exhaling with relief, as I am.

As Susan serves the cake, I realize it is a smaller group this year. I've been paying attention to Janni, playing with her because she won't play with anyone else, and didn't notice. That explains the pizza situation. Last year people stayed for hours, long after the cake and the presents. This year, some have already left. Looking around, I realize that Lynn and the twins are gone, too.

CHAPTER TWO

October 2006

Janni's IQ is 146.

This can't be right. I was expecting it to be higher, a lot higher. I was expecting Albert Einstein IQ or Stephen Hawking IQ (although neither man ever submitted to an IQ test).

I am sitting in the office of Heidi Yellen, a therapist who specializes in autism spectrum disorders. As Janni's behavior has changed, more of our friends have started bringing up autism. Besides the new antisocial behavior, Janni can't stop moving her hands, which everybody takes as "stimming," one of the predominant signs of autism. Janni's pediatrician referred us to her, "just to rule it out." I didn't want to take Janni. Autism is the diagnosis du jour, just like hyperactivity used to be when I was a kid. I still resent that the rest of the world seems more concerned with Janni's behavior than with her intelligence, but I am getting tired of constantly hearing people suggest it. So I go, terrified Janni will be diagnosed autistic and that that will derail her future.

However, to my great pleasure and surprise, the first thing Heidi wants to do is give Janni an IQ test. This is what I want, proof of Janni's genius, to refute those who suggest there is something wrong with her.

Except that 146 isn't what I'm looking for. I want a number so high it allows me to explain away and even justify Janni's increasing disengagement from kids her age and the preference she has for her imaginary friends. I want to be able to say, when Janni does something antisocial, "Well, she has an IQ of 280."

"So 146," I say to Heidi, then look up to see Janni sneaking behind Heidi to her computer. "Janni! Don't play with Heidi's computer!"

"I'm bored," Janni complains as she roughly punches the keys on Heidi's computer.

Susan isn't getting off the couch. I think she's still in shock, too. The trade-off is there's nobody to keep Janni engaged while I try to comprehend this. Then again, it's not like Susan can keep Janni engaged anyway.

"I just need a few minutes, Janni. This is important."

I watch Janni to see whether she's going to give in or bolt from the office. She has a grin on her face that disturbs me because it alters her expression, making her look calculating and manipulative. But what really bothers me is that it doesn't look like Janni at all. If I believed in demonic possession, I would swear that in these moments she's possessed.

Janni is sneaking back to the computer.

"Janni." Heidi turns to her. "I asked you before not to play with my computer. I have important files on it."

"I'm working," Janni replies, the same twisted smile on her face, still randomly punching away at the keyboard.

"Janni, she asked you not to touch her computer! We have to respect other people's things."

"Here, you can play with this." Heidi hands her a toy.

Heidi turns back to me. "You need to look at the percentages. On the next page."

I nervously look away from Janni, knowing that toy will only hold her interest for a few seconds. I turn the page of the document Heidi has given me. I see things like "*Verbal >99.9%.*"

"This is why I needed you to come in instead of just mailing the results," Heidi goes on. "There are things I need to explain."

"I want to go," Janni whines.

"We're going to go. I just need a second."

"If you look at all her percentages," Heidi goes on, "some of them, such as verbal, are even greater than ninety-nine percent."

She points to one of the marks that show >99.9%. "This means that she reached the maximum the test can calculate."

"What?" I ask, distracted as Janni breaks for the office door. "Janni! Come over here. We're almost done." I stand up, terrified Janni is going to run, which she does. "No" and "Stay here" have no meaning. If we don't go where she wants, Janni will literally just walk out the door. I only have a few more seconds to get as much information as I can. "What does that mean exactly?"

"It means she broke the test. One-fifty is as high as the Stanford-Binet Five test goes. She's at 146, and that was without any writing. I couldn't get her to do any writing."

"Yeah, neither can we," I say, holding on to Janni's arm, keeping her next to me as she tries to run again.

"She knows how to write, but gets frustrated because she can't write like a computer. She screams and tears up the paper," Susan adds.

"There could be some OCD," Heidi says, relenting. "But here's the issue. Mentally, she's between ten and eleven. That is where all your problems are going to come from."

I let this sink in: *mental capacity of a ten- or eleven-year-old*. Janni is four. Her mind is older than her body. She is angry because she is mentally older than she looks, but all everybody other than Susan and I sees is a little kid.

"So what do we do now that we know?" I ask.

"She needs to go to a gifted school."

Yes! That is what I want, so maybe Janni will find others like her.

"Can you recommend any?"

"Mirman."

I sigh. Mirman is a school for highly gifted kids. We've already contacted them. But there are two problems. One, all kids must be potty-trained and Janni is still wearing Pull-Ups. She knows how to go but refuses to do it in the potty. She runs around without a diaper for hours. When she has to go, she gets a diaper, puts it on, does her business, then takes it off and puts it in the trash. There is no bribing her, for the same reason that punishing her doesn't work. At one point, trying to get her to behave, I took away all her toys except for her favorite stuffed bear, Hero, which she sleeps with. I would never take him. Her toys sat up above the kitchen cabinets for weeks and Janni didn't care. The only things she really cares about are her imaginary friends, and I can't take them away.

Mirman also requires an "entrance interview." In my mind, I can see how that would play out. The principal walks in and says, "Hello, January," and Janni screams, "I'm not January!" And that would be the end of that.

"We have already talked to Mirman," I say to Heidi. "They won't take her unless she is potty-trained."

"Well, maybe when they see these numbers they'll change their mind."

I have my doubts. Mirman seems pretty strict about their rules.

I am convinced that all Janni needs is kids like her, kids with her genius, and everything will be fine, but stupid rules prevent her from reaching her potential.

"You just have to keep trying," Heidi replies. "There is no other option. She has to go to Mirman. She will not make it in regular school."

I lose my grip, and Janni flies out the door.

CHAPTER THREE

February 2007

W here are we going?" Janni asks. "I want pizza."

"We're going to Violet's birthday party." I grit my teeth, knowing what's coming.

"I don't like Violet!"

I sigh.

"Janni, she's a nice girl."

"I hate her," she says, like she's pointing out it's a sunny day. There is no animosity in her voice, which is why I don't believe her.

"Why do you hate her? Hate is such a strong emotion, Janni. We reserve hate for people who really hurt us. Violet's never hurt you."

"I still don't like her."

Janni doesn't have many friends left, but I cling to hope with Violet. Violet is a smart girl. I can dismiss how Janni treats other kids when they're not on her "level," but that's not the case with Violet.

"Why not?" I press, desperate for her not to alienate Violet.

"She doesn't like dogs."

"Did you ask her?"

"No."

"How do you know she doesn't like dogs?"

"I just know."

"How do you know?" I persist.

"400 tells me."

I consider reminding her that 400 isn't real, but that never works, so I ask, "And how does 400 know?"

Janni shrugs. "I don't know. She just does."

"Violet's not a thirteen, Janni. She is smart. She has to be pretty close to a twenty."

Janni is silent for a moment. "I'm a twenty-five now."

Deep inside me, the fear that I refuse to acknowledge stirs. She's raising her "number." "When did you become a twenty-five?"

"I just am."

This bothers me. Every time I think we may have found a friend closer to Janni's number, she raises it, like she's deliberately trying to create distance between herself and everybody else.

"Well, just promise me that you won't tell Violet that you don't like her."

"I am going to tell her that."

This catches me by surprise. It's like she is tattling on herself. Even if she planned to, why not lie to me? That would be the logical thing to do.

"Remember what Mommy said about not saying anything if you can't say anything nice?" I reply.

"Violet doesn't get my imagination."

I sigh. *I know, Janni.* The imagination of kids her age seems to be limited to pretending to be princesses and crap like that. None of them are capable of conceiving of an entirely separate world like Janni is with Calilini. I hate seeing Janni try to communicate her world to other children. Every time it happens, I grow more afraid inside, fearing that one day she'll just stop trying.

SARA, VIOLET'S MOTHER, opens the front door to greet us, and I hand over Violet's present.

Violet runs up to Janni and extends her arms, stepping forward to hug her, but Janni shrugs her off like a coat, her head down, unwilling to make eye contact.

It's already starting, just like always.

"Janni, tell Violet 'Happy birthday,'" I command.

"I hate you," Janni says to Violet.

"Janni! What did I say?" I refuse to look up for fear of what I will see in Sara's face. Instead, I turn to Violet.

"I'm sorry, Violet. Don't take it personally. Janni says that to everyone." It occurs to me how ridiculous that sounds. I just told a five-year-old not to take something personally. I have gotten so used to talking to Janni like an adult that I forget other kids her age can't understand.

Violet stands there, not sure what to do.

"Well, we are glad you could come, Janni," Sara says politely, but I can feel her trying to brush off Janni's rudeness like it's no big deal. And this worries me, too. If I can feel it, I worry Janni can, too. I want to protect her from the judgment of others, not keep exposing her to it. I get angry at Susan for making us come to this party.

"Do you have pizza?" is all Janni asks.

"No, I'm sorry. There's no pizza," Sara replies apologetically.

There goes my only chance of keeping her here for any length of time. The only reason I was even able to get her to come was by telling her there would be pizza.

"But we have plenty of other food," Sara adds sweetly, as if Janni is just any other little girl.

I look over at the spread. The food seems more for adults than for kids; bagels and cream cheese, veggie platters. Nothing Janni will eat.

I AM PUSHING Janni on the swing set in Violet's backyard while the other girls are in the house playing a game.

Some other parents are talking on the patio, holding their paper plates with veggies and dip, cheese and crackers. I feel a tinge of bitterness. They can let their kids run wild, never having to worry about their son or daughter saying or doing something hurtful to another child.

Hovering below the other parents, waiting for any food that might fall, is a small white dog. So much for Janni's conviction that Violet doesn't like dogs.

"Janni, are you sure you don't want to go in and play?" I expect she'll refuse, but I ask anyway because I am tired of us always being on the fringes. "It looks like fun."

"No."

"What if I play, too?"

"No."

I resign myself to the continued isolation and push her on the swing.

"I'm ready to get off," Janni announces, so I grab one of the swing's ropes and slow it down.

She gets off and runs back inside the house.

I follow, moving as quickly as I can through the maze of other parents, trying not to bump into any of them. I have to catch up to Janni so I can cut off any conflict that might come between her and the rest of the world.

Thankfully, and a bit to my surprise, Janni has stopped in the living room to watch Sara leading Violet and the other girls in a game of Red Rover.

"Hey, Janni!" Sara spots us. "You want to play?"

"It's a fun game," I add, hoping the game will lure Janni in.

"No. I just wanna watch."

I don't know why she wants to watch and not play. When she was eighteen months old, she would walk up to other toddlers and ask them their names, even though most of them didn't yet talk. She was always interested in other children. Now they can talk and she's not interested.

I glance down and realize Janni is not beside me anymore. She slipped away and I didn't even notice. My first instinct is to scan the kids, hoping Janni has joined in the game after all, but no, she isn't among the happy, laughing girls. Wishful thinking. Maybe she went out to the backyard again? I go back outside to the swing, but she isn't there.

Panic is rising inside of me. This is what she always does. When she wants to leave, she just goes. I am terrified she might have just walked out the door. She's done it before.

I start searching the house, room by room. Finally, I go into Violet's room. The blinds are pulled and the corners of the room are filled with shadows. It takes a moment for my eyes to adjust. Then I see Janni, down on the floor, pulling Violet's stuffed animals off her bed and lining them up.

Violet comes into the room behind me. At first I think she just came to get something, because her friends aren't with her. She has plenty of other girls who actually want to be her friend. Why waste her time with a girl who tells her she hates her?

But to my surprise, she sits down next to Janni.

"Hi," she says to Janni.

Janni ignores Violet like she isn't even there.

Violet takes a stuffed lion out of the line Janni is building. The lion. Leo. Janni's astrological sign.

"I call this one Mr. Lion," Violet says to Janni.

Janni grabs the lion back. "That's 60."

"Why not 'Mr. 60 the Lion'?" I suggest to Janni.

"No. He's 60."

"Can't he be both?" I ask hopefully. This is different. Violet is different. She is really trying. *Please, Janni,* I think to myself, *just give a little.*

"No," Janni answers.

Violet picks up a doll. "This is my favorite. Her name is Elle."

Janni looks askew at the doll. "That's 11." She takes the doll from Violet.

But Violet doesn't get angry. She leans in next to Janni, so close their hair is touching. Violet's short brown hair looks so neatly combed next to Janni's tangled mess of curls that she won't let us brush anymore.

Janni is hunched over the stuffed animals, talking to herself.

Something about this sight looks familiar, but I can't place it. And then it hits me with a force that makes me shiver. In the twilight of the room, huddled over, Violet next to her, trying to reach her, trying to be her friend, Janni looks like a shut-in. She is Laura in *The Glass Menagerie,* lost in her own world. I feel a sob rising in my throat, but I fight it down. No, I am being overdramatic. This is just a stage. Janni will outgrow this.

SUSAN IS JUST getting out of her car, having come straight from work, as Sara opens the door to let us out.

Susan smiles and waves to Violet, who is standing at the door to say good-bye, like the well-behaved hostess she has been trained to be. I am barging out the door, following Janni.

"Where are you going?" Susan asks me, as Janni and I pass her.

"I need to feed Janni," I snarl. "She's hungry and there was no pizza."

"Yes, I'm sorry," Sara says, like nothing is happening. "I didn't know that's what Janni wanted."

"She is a very picky eater." There goes Susan again, always explaining everything. Then to me, "What about the cake? Have they had the cake yet?"

"The cake is still an hour away. I can't keep Janni here that long. I need to get her fed."

I am furious at Susan. I refuse to get angry with Janni. This isn't her fault. She never wanted to come to this party in the first place.

"She should at least have some cake," Susan protests.

"I'm getting her out of here," I say, crossing the street to our car, Janni already ahead of me. "I never should've brought her."

"I want pizza," Janni adds.

Susan is rushing after us as I open the car door and climb in.

"What happened? Why are you so angry?"

I turn on her.

"You're torturing her."

Susan looks confused.

"What are you talking about?"

"What you are doing to her, forcing her to come to birthday parties and taking her to playdates, it's torture."

"I'm only trying to find her friends," Susan answers.

"I'm tired of it," I yell. "I'm tired of you always insisting that she will get along with this child or that child, and every damn time I actually fall for it, hoping you're right, but it's always the same. I just watched Violet trying so hard to connect with Janni, and Janni just ignored her. I won't do it anymore."

"Fine," Susan answers. "It sounds more like you can't handle it. I'll take her."

"No," I hiss at her. "I am not going to let you keep exposing her to people that will only make her feel like a freak! She's brilliant!"

"I know she's brilliant!" Susan fires back.

"That's not the point! Janni's IQ is higher than 99.9 percent of the population. That means out of six billion people, Janni is smarter than all but six million of them!"

"That's still a lot."

"They could be anywhere in the world! Do you know what the odds are of finding any of them?"

"We have to keep trying," Susan answers.

"No, we don't. We can leave her in peace."

"So what I am supposed to do? Stop trying to find her friends?"

"Exactly." I slam the car door on Susan and drive off with Janni.

CHAPTER FOUR

December 16, 2007

The blinds are open and darkness is descending quickly around us as the green LED lights of the fetal heart monitor blink at me. I see our son's heartbeat as a staggered yellow line crossing the monitor screen. His name will be Bodhi, the tree under which Siddhartha Gautama was sitting when he achieved enlightenment and became the Buddha. We aren't Buddhists or even religious, but we hope that our son can bring peace to Janni just as the shade of the Bodhi Tree brought comfort to the Buddha.

In the light shining in from the hospital corridor, I can barely make out Susan's head. I'm not sure if she is asleep. I know I should be with her to welcome Bodhi coming into this world, but I can't stop worrying about Janni. She needs me. I can sense it.

I feel for my cell phone in my pocket and fight the desire to call and check in. I have to let this go. I have to trust that my dad can handle her.

"I wonder how your dad is doing with Janni," Susan comments from the darkness, startling me. Even she is thinking about Janni, despite waiting for the anesthesiologist to come and insert the epidural needle into her spine.

"I'm sure they're probably fine," I say, trying to convince myself as much as Susan. Janni has never been apart from both of us at the same time until tonight.

We fall silent, listening to the beep of Bodhi's heartbeat. It's hard for me to believe that just ten months ago, I had no intention of ever having another child. Susan had been talking about it for a while, reminding me that her "time was running out."

But that was not why I finally agreed to a second child. I wanted Bodhi for one reason and one reason only: because Janni said she wanted a sibling. Bodhi is the biggest gamble I have ever made in my life. For five years, we've been trying to find another child who would "get" Janni's imagination, and failed. So this is my last-ditch attempt. If I can't find a child whom Janni can relate to, maybe I can create one?

"I can't believe I'm about to say this," I speak quietly from the dark, "but I actually hope Bodhi is just like Janni."

"I know."

"I mean it. I would go through this all again. The total lack of sleep and the having to constantly stimulate him."

"We won't have to do that. Bodhi will have what Janni didn't have, an older sibling."

I chuckle.

"Knowing our luck, this one will probably sleep." The smile dies on my lips. "But if I have to do it all over again, I will, if it will mean Janni has somebody like her."

"I feel the same way." Susan's arm reaches out for me.

I stand up and take it.

"You should probably call your dad and check on Janni," Susan says to me.

"Okay." I go out into the hall and call my father.

"Is everything okay?" I ask when he answers the phone.

"Well, we went to the mall, to that play area, but she didn't want to stay very long. She tried to run off."

I close my eyes. This is exactly what I was afraid of.

"So where are you going now?" I ask.

"We're going to take her to dinner."

I look over at Susan. Even in the shadows, I can see her eyes, nervous. I make a decision.

"Come back to the hospital and pick me up."

"Michael, it's fine. You need to be with Susan," my dad tells me.

"Susan's fine. Bodhi's not coming tonight anyway. I can go for a few hours."

"You sure?"

"Yes."

"Okay," he agrees, a little too quickly. "We'll pick you up in front of the hospital in ten minutes."

I hang up and turn back to Susan.

"Everything okay? How is Janni?" I can hear the anxiety in her voice.

"Dad took her to the mall, but she got bored and wanted to leave. Now they're going to dinner."

"How do you think she is doing with him?"

I sigh. "He can't handle her."

"Did something happen?" she asks, her voice cracking.

"No, I don't think so. But I better go with them to dinner."

Susan falls silent for second. She knows. We both had a strong feeling this might happen. Of course, we wanted to believe Janni would do okay without us, but deep down we knew. We couldn't trust anybody else to stimulate Janni to the same extent we do.

"Are you going to be okay?" I ask. "I'll only be gone for a little while."

"It's not like I haven't been through this before," she says, trying to sound cavalier, but I can hear the disappointment in her voice.

This is wrong. I am abandoning my wife at the time she needs me most. But Janni needs me more. Susan will have the hospital staff. Janni has no one.

I take Susan's hand, threaded with IVs, in mine.

"Let me go with her to dinner, get her down, and then I will be back. I promise."

"I know. I feel better that you'll be with her anyway." Susan cranes her neck for a kiss, and I bend down to meet her.

MY DAD, WHO flew in from Arizona, rented a boat of a car. I get into the backseat with Janni. Even in the dark I can see her eyes. She has gone to that place inside her mind where nothing out here matters to her. I need to say something silly to snap her out of it, but I can't. I shouldn't even have to be here. I should be back with Susan. I resent my father. If he would only play with her like I do. Why is it so hard for everyone else? I've been doing this for five years and my dad can't even handle an hour.

My dad starts asking me questions about how Susan is doing.

"She's fine," I answer curtly. "How were things at the mall?"

"Well," he begins. I can see his face in the rearview mirror. "We had some problems. Janni kicked me."

I exhale sharply and turn my head to look out the window. Normally, when this type of thing happens, I make a show of chastising Janni, but in my mind I justify it as part of her struggle with the world that sees her as just an ordinary child. But this is my father. I can't let this go.

"Janni! Why did you do that?" I ask, turning to her. I am scared. I don't trust my dad to put up with this, even though she is his only grandchild. I want to believe that because he is blood he will hang on, but I sense he is on the edge, after only an hour.

I hear the sound of a foot striking something solid.

"Janni, don't do that," Dad says. "It's distracting for me."

Janni is kicking the back of my father's seat. I don't see any anger. It is like she is swinging her legs in the breeze.

"Janni, Grandpa needs to drive," I tell her. I hear my own voice in my ears. I am begging. I know where this is going.

Janni keeps swinging her legs into the back of my dad's seat.

"Janni, stop that!" he commands, like he used to do with me. Whenever I heard that tone from him as a kid, I stopped immediately. That tone scared me. It still does and I'm an adult. But Janni is not me. The stern voice of authority means nothing to her. I can see her eyes. The "this is a funny game" look has returned.

She keeps kicking. I feel paralyzed, not sure what to do. I could yell at her, too, but that would only make her do it more.

She keeps kicking the back of my father's seat.

"Janni! For the last time, I said 'Stop it!'"

But Janni is not going to stop. "For the last time" means nothing to her, because she has nothing to lose. I need to distract her, get her mind on something else other than kicking my dad's seat, but I can't think of anything.

Janni continues to kick.

"Janni!" my father roars. He takes his right hand off the steering wheel and reaches around. I feel like I am watching a plane crash in slow motion. He lightly spanks her on her knee.

My dad settles back into his seat, thinking he has solved the problem. What he doesn't know, what he can't see in the dark of the backseat, is that I have unbuckled my seat belt and am leaning across the seat, putting my full weight on Janni's legs because she is still trying to kick the back of his seat.

CHAPTER FIVE

December 22, 2007

We cannot let Bodhi make a sound. In the three days since we brought him home, we have come to fear the slightest peep out of him. As soon as he begins to stir, even before he opens his eyes, we put a pacifier or bottle into his mouth.

Every few minutes, I come over to Bodhi's crib. He is still asleep. I check for any signs he might be close to waking up.

I look over at Janni, a few feet away, standing in front of the TV set, so close there's no way she could see the entire picture, yet she's totally absorbed by the show.

I return to the kitchen, where I am forever washing Bodhi's baby bottles. There are already five full bottles waiting in the fridge, but I want to make sure more are ready.

The volume on the TV is rising. I run over to see the volume bar moving across the screen, the numbers climbing to 59, maximum volume. Steve from *Blue's Clues* booms around the apartment.

"Janni, turn it down!" I hiss, turning the volume back down, looking nervously over at Bodhi, afraid the deafening noise will wake him up. He's been asleep for four hours and he'll be waking up soon. I don't want to speed up the process.

Janni turns the volume all the way back up again.

"Janni, that is too loud." I rush to turn it down again.

"But I can't hear it!" Janni suddenly erupts, turning it back up.

"How can you not hear it? You're right in front of it."

"I can't hear it," she complains again.

A weak cry comes from the couch. Bodhi has been rudely returned to the world.

"Susan!" I yell, breaking for the kitchen. The countdown to detonation has begun.

"I'm coming!" Susan leaps out of bed, where she was resting, and runs into the living room like I'd yelled *"Fire!"*

She gathers Bodhi up in her arms, while I fling open the refrigerator and grab a ready-made bottle of formula.

"I can't hear over Bodhi's crying!" Janni screams out, never taking her eyes off the TV, even though she's seen this episode a million times before.

We are running out of time to defuse the proverbial bomb. I run back to Susan with the bottle. She wearily puts it into Bodhi's mouth. He grimaces and wails louder, formula running from his mouth. Shit! I was so panicked I forgot to warm the bottle up to room temperature. Janni never cared, but Bodhi is extremely sensitive to temperature.

"Bodhi!" Janni's shriek pierces the room, never turning from the TV. "Stop crying!"

Her scream only makes him cry louder. I can hear the fear in his cry. He doesn't know what is happening. It is not supposed to be like this. This should be a safe environment. I rush back to the kitchen and put the bottle in the microwave.

"Stop crying!" Janni puts her hands over her ears, even though the TV is the loudest thing in the apartment.

"Janni, if it is bothering you, go into the bedroom," Susan says soothingly.

"I'm watching this!"

"We have a TV in the bedroom," Susan reminds her.

"I'm watching this!" she repeats, as if the request is unreasonable.

I pull the bottle out of the microwave and rush it over to Bodhi. "Nobody likes the sound of a crying baby, Janni. We're wired to hate it," I say, trying to teach her as a means of distracting her from Bodhi's crying. "It's evolution's way of making sure we take care of our young."

Bodhi opens his mouth up, eager for the nipple, but then breaks off screaming again. It is too hot now. I overshot. I didn't have time to warm it for a few seconds, check it, and warm it again.

"Stop crying!" Janni shouts over the top of him and then unleashes one of her earsplitting screams. Bodhi's crying goes up in volume.

"Janni!" I yell, racing back to the kitchen, pulling one of the half-clean bottles out of the sink and rinsing it out. I am going to have to make new formula that will be room temperature. It's faster than trying to warm one of the remaining bottles in the fridge. "Screaming at him will only make him cry harder."

"But he's crying!" Janni screams, her hands over her ears.

I try to keep my hand from shaking while measuring scoops of formula. Time is almost up. We only have a few seconds left. I am so scared that it is a struggle to get the nipple on the bottle correctly.

"Janni, no!" Susan cries out, panicked. I look up to see her arm go out in protection. She jerks Bodhi in her arms, as the remote control goes flying past. The abrupt movement scares Bodhi even more.

Janni just threw the remote control at Bodhi.

"Janni, no throwing!" I shout. Time is up. The firing mechanism has been triggered. It is too late now to stop Janni from going off. "Go into the other room now!" I command.

Janni calmly walks around the coffee table that separates her from Susan and Bodhi. Susan starts to get up, recoiling, twisting to shield Bodhi. Janni reaches up and drives her fist into Susan's stomach, just below Bodhi's dangling legs.

I have seen this every day since we brought Bodhi home, but it still paralyzes me for a moment, the sight of my daughter attacking my wife and son.

Susan turns her back to Janni, trying to shield Bodhi. Janni's fist comes down on her back so hard I can hear the "thud" from across the room. Susan stumbles forward. I watch her twist in mid-fall, turning Bodhi away from the oncoming couch. Susan lands hard on the couch, crying out. Janni pushes past her legs, coming on, silent, totally devoid of emotion, totally focused on her hitting. Susan rotates away.

"Help me!" she calls to me in desperation.

I finally snap out of my temporary paralysis and cross over to Janni, grabbing her arm in midair.

"Janni, stop that! No hitting!"

Janni doesn't respond. I feel her arm pulling against my hand. She keeps pulling for several seconds before she seems to realize something is holding on to her arm. She turns to me. Her other fist rises and comes down in my stomach.

The strength of the impact catches me off guard, pushing all the air out of my lungs as her fist buries itself in my solar plexus.

"Janni, you need to stop . . . ," I say, as calmly as I can manage. I need to stay calm and maybe it might rub off on her. I grab her other arm, holding them both firmly, but careful to make sure I don't hurt her. My goal is just to immobilize her and wait it out.

She kicks me in the shin. Hard. She is wearing no shoes. How can that not have hurt her foot? I wonder.

I have to get her out of here, away from Bodhi, who is still screaming in terror. I pick her up off the ground, embracing her in a bear hug, and turn for the bedroom. I feel her fist slam into the side of my head, sending a shock wave of pain through my temple. She continues hitting me in the head, punching me as hard as she can.

I reposition her in my arms to get a firmer grip so I don't drop her when she hits me again. She is still my daughter, and I am more concerned about her getting hurt than me. I grit my teeth so I can take the pain. I can't grab her hands without putting her down, and if I do, I know she will tear loose and go after Bodhi again.

I don't tell her to stop. There is no point. This has happened several times a day since we brought Bodhi home. I get Janni into the bedroom and onto the bed, where I can hold her until this passes. And it always does. This explosion of violence subsides as quickly as it came. I don't have time to worry about what caused it. All I am focused on is just surviving these next few minutes without any of us getting hurt.

"Let me go!" she screams, thrashing against me. I lie next to her, holding her arms down.

"Are you going to hurt Bodhi?" I ask.

She stops thrashing and looks up at me. I feel a rush of hope. "If you tell me you won't try to hurt Bodhi, I can let you go," I tell her.

"I have to hurt Bodhi," she answers in a voice like she is being forced to hurt him.

"No, you don't. You may *feel* like you have to, but you don't."

She nods. "I do have to. . . . I want to."

I'm confused. Does she want to hurt him because she *has* to or because she *wants* to? I would rather it be the former. I don't want to believe that she wants to hurt her baby brother.

"Janni, just tell me you won't try to hurt him and I can let you go," I say out of desperation.

"I am going to hurt him," she replies, very matter-of-factly.

She is being irrational. The rational thing to do, the "smart" thing to do, would be to lie to me and tell me she won't hurt Bodhi, even if it isn't true, just so I would let her go. I can't understand why she insists on telling me the truth. It is not a truth I want to hear.

She kicks her legs into my side. I have her arms still pinned, so she's gone to her next weapon. I place one leg over both her legs, trying to hold them down while still keeping my weight off her. I weigh one hundred and fifty pounds more than she does and I don't want to hurt her. This is not about punishment. This is about hanging on until she calms down.

She is twisting her head back and forth, her eyes closed. "You're hurting me!"

"No, I am not, Janni," I reply calmly, even though I check my grip to make sure I'm not holding her any tighter than I have to, just enough to keep her limbs immobile. "I am just holding you. Now, are you going to stop trying to hit Bodhi?"

"No!"

Her answer flusters me.

"Janni, just tell me you won't hurt Bodhi and I will let you go."

"I want to hurt him!"

"He hasn't done anything to you!"

"Yes, he is!" she says, as though he's hurting her at this exact moment.

"But he isn't, and never has." I am desperate for a reason, anything that will explain this sudden violence. "Just tell me what you are angry about, Janni."

"He's crying," she answers.

"Babies cry," I reply. "Nobody likes the sound of a baby crying, but he won't cry forever."

"Yes, he will."

Her answer makes no sense. *You understand so much, Janni. Why can't you understand this, too?*

"No, he won't."

"I can't take his crying!"

"Then walk away! Go into the other room."

"I can still hear him!" she cries. I pause, listening. I can't hear him. Susan has obviously calmed him down again, or he must be eating.

I feel teeth closing down on my chin.

"Ahhhhh!" I cry out. I didn't expect her to bite, but I realize now that with her arms and legs pinned, she is using the last weapon at her disposal. I glance down. She looks like a wild animal attached to my chin. I can feel her teeth going through my flesh. "Janni, Janni, Janni. . . . Let go, sweetie."

She is biting down harder. This is the most physical pain I have ever felt in my life. Automatically, my arms let go of hers and move to my face. Despite her being free now, she's still biting down on my chin. I pull back, but this only makes my pain worse. Tears form at the edge of my eyes. I fight the intense desire to pull free.

This is not my daughter. This can't be my daughter. My real daughter makes me fish drowning bees out of the pool. The person hurting me is just in her body. I just have to ride this out until it lets go of her. I steel myself to take whatever pain I have to take.

Finally, she lets go. I lift my head out of the range of her mouth. Her mouth hangs open, her head up, like I've seen crocodiles do on TV. She is not making eye contact with me. She glares at my chin like she is considering eating it.

"Janni, that hurt," I say, as if she had just bumped me. I am trying to gently remind her that she is inflicting pain. Maybe if she realizes this it will make her stop.

"You're hurting me!" she cries, thrashing her head back and forth. I don't get this at all. I'm not even touching her anymore. Abruptly, I feel the sting of fingernails digging into my forehead.

"Janni . . ."

I close my eyes as she drags her nails down the length of my face. I can feel my skin slicing open and the sting of blood meeting air.

Her hands detach from my face.

I breathe heavily, my face stinging sharply.

I roll off her, gingerly touching the scratches on my face. Hopefully, she has gotten all her violence out of her system. I sit on the edge of the bed watching her, ready to grab her again if she goes after Bodhi, adrenaline making me only dully aware of my own pain.

She looks over at me. "I'm hungry."

"Okay," I say. It is over, I realize. That is how it is. The violence leaves as quickly as it comes. "What do you want?"

Janni looks around and finally meets my eyes. I see no recognition of what she has done. It is like this never happened.

"Do we have any mac 'n' cheese?" she asks, rubbing her hands together excitedly.

CHAPTER SIX

Christmas Week, 2007

I pull into a parking space outside my therapist's office. My appointment starts now, but I need a cigarette.

I started seeing my therapist, Tom, the previous spring for the unresolved anger issues over my mother. I could forgive her for padlocking the refrigerator so we wouldn't "overeat," even though it made me so hungry I stole handfuls of dry dog food out of our dog's food bag. Ironically, my mother confessed that she'd been doing the same thing. So why was she padlocking the refrigerator?

I could even forgive her for chasing me out of the house with a butcher knife, because she told me later that she thought I was her father trying to rape her.

But what I couldn't forgive was that after my parents divorced and I chose to live with my father at fifteen, she never tried to see me again. So I'd come to Tom to try and find a way to deal with my mother's abandonment.

But I haven't come to talk about my mother today, because nothing in my past seems to matter anymore. Now I fear the future. I am terrified that if Janni ever manages to reach Bodhi during one of her episodes, she will kill him. I wouldn't have believed that a five-year-old could be this violent if I hadn't been on the receiving end of it. I have scratches and bruises all over me. My entire body aches. But I am thirty-one years old. Bodhi is a newborn. One punch to his body could be life-and-death for him.

My hands shake as I light another cigarette. My nerves are raw. This is the worst fear I have ever known in my life. I look at Bodhi through the tinted rear window. He is still asleep. I brought him because Susan and I have already instituted a new rule, a week into Bodhi's life: Neither one of us ever leaves the other alone with both Janni and Bodhi. At all times when our children are together, one of us must take care of Bodhi, protecting him, and the other must be ready to block Janni.

By the time I reach Tom's office, I'm nearly fifteen minutes late and lugging the still-sleeping Bodhi in his car seat. Tom is sitting in his chair, his door open, but I knock to let him know I'm here.

"Hi, Tom. Sorry I'm so late."

He looks up. "I saw you through the window down in the parking lot. I was wondering when you were coming up." There is no annoyance in his voice, only concern. "Is everything okay?"

I hold up Bodhi's car seat.

"Is it okay if I bring my son in?" I ask. If he says no, then I have no choice but to leave.

He looks down at Bodhi, a look of surprise on his face. I'm not sure whether he is surprised to see me bringing my newborn out so soon or if he is just shocked that I brought one of my children to my therapy session.

"He should just sleep," I say. "He's not like Janni. He sleeps."

He sticks his finger in his ear, which he always does when I say something that throws him.

"Ah, yeah, sure, I guess, as long as it's not going to be a regular thing. I don't mind, but I wouldn't want to disturb Kate." Kate is the therapist in the next office.

I sit down, placing Bodhi's car seat on the floor below me.

"Then I don't know that I will be able to come anymore."

Tom's brow furrows. "What's going on?"

I pour out to Tom everything that has been happening since Bodhi was born. As I listen to myself, I think it sounds insane.

"I don't know what is happening to Janni," I finally conclude. "You're a psychologist. What do you think?"

Tom exhales. "I don't work with children, so I am not the best person to say, but from what you describe it sounds like she is pretty disturbed."

Pretty disturbed. That's not what I was expecting to hear. I have to believe there must be a rational explanation for this. I was expecting him to tell me that he has heard of this before and it is a phase that can be treated through therapy. But that's not what he said. He just said *pretty disturbed*, in the way people say the word "cancer."

TOM GETS US in to see Kate, his office mate and a child psychologist, in less than three days.

When Kate, a curly-black-haired woman in her sixties, comes out of her office, she's clearly surprised to see all of us there. She was expecting just Susan and me for the first visit. But who could take care of Janni and Bodhi and keep Bodhi safe from Janni? We had no choice but to bring both kids.

Janni tries to run into her office.

"No, January," Kate tells her. "I need to speak to your mommy and daddy first."

I instinctively flinch, knowing what is coming.

"I'm not January!" Janni screams, turning and hitting Kate, who recoils.

I grab Janni, pulling her back. "Sorry, she doesn't like her name or any variation of it."

Kate looks shocked, which bothers me. She is a child psychologist, an expert in child behavior. How can she be shocked by this?

"I'm 76," Janni says.

"Will she play out here for a few minutes," Kate asks, regaining her composure, "if I get her some crayons and paper?"

I look at her like she's insane.

"That won't work," I reply, trying to hide the frustration in my voice. I don't want Kate to see me get angry and think I'm the problem. "One of us will have to go in at a time while the other stays out here with Janni," I say. "You go first," I tell Susan. "I'll stay out here with her."

WE USE BLOCKS to build things. First a house, then . . . "Look, Janni. I made a slide."

"That's a rat slide." Janni places the imaginary Wednesday the Rat on the block slide. "There you go, Wednesday." Janni pauses. "She likes it." She looks up at me, genuinely happy, as if there were a chance her imaginary friend wouldn't like it.

She looks away at the closed door to Kate's office, and I know she's already lost interest. Like it or not, we're finished with the blocks.

"I wanna go in."

"Soon, Janni."

"There's nothing to do here!"

"Do you want to build another house?" I ask, even though I know she won't want to. I look at the clock on my cell phone. Less than ten minutes has passed since Susan went in. I look around the office, desperate for something else I can use to buy a few more minutes.

I spot a *National Geographic* magazine on the end table, one that has the pandas of China. Janni likes animals.

"Janni, do you want to see some pandas?"

But Janni's already opening Kate's door, so I toss the magazine aside, rushing over.

"Sorry," I say to Kate as I follow Janni in, "I couldn't keep her out there anymore."

Kate looks surprised at us barging in. Again, this bothers me. It is Janni's behavior we are here for, after all.

"That's okay," Kate says, quickly recovering. "We were about ready for her anyway."

Janni is moving through the office, searching for something to engage her mind. I am her shadow, right behind her, ready for anything. I see some board games but no toys. And this is the office of a child psychologist?

Janni turns to Kate. "Where are your toys?"

"I don't have too many toys. I suppose I should get more, but most of the kids I see are a little older than you," she replies. "I have some paper and crayons. Do you want to draw?"

I hide my frustration, knowing this won't work. But to my surprise Janni agrees.

"What are you going to draw?" Kate asks Janni, sitting her down at the desk near her.

"Wednesday, my pet rat."

"You have a pet rat named Wednesday?"

"I have seven rats," Janni answers, drawing furiously. I watch over her shoulder. She is scribbling circles within circles, like how a hurricane looks on a weather map.

Susan pipes in. "They're not real rats. She has a lot of imaginary friends."

"They're not imaginary," Janni answers, with just a little irritation.

"You have a pet dog, Honey," Susan prompts.

"I don't like Honey," Janni answers, with no particular venom. This is new. I've never heard that before. She loves our dog.

Janni finishes drawing and hands the paper to Kate.

"You're done already?" Kate asks, clearly surprised.

Janni nods, pointing to the mass of scribbles. "That's Wednesday."

"Do you want to draw me another picture?" Kate asks, but Janni is already moving on.

Susan hands Kate Janni's IQ results. "Here are her IQ results," she says. "She tested with a 146 IQ at four years old. We don't know if her genius is related to what is going on."

"Janni?" Kate asks. "How do you feel about Bodhi?"

"I hate him," Janni answers, not looking over, still searching the office.

"Why do you hate him?" Kate asks.

"Because he cries," Janni answers, disinterestedly.

Kate turns to me. "Older children often have a hard time adapting when a sibling comes along."

I am getting increasingly annoyed.

"You don't understand. This isn't a normal tantrum we are talking about. The only way I can describe it is like Regan from *The Exorcist*. One minute she is her sweet, normal self, and the next she is literally trying to scratch my eyes out. Then she is back to normal like nothing happened. She doesn't sulk or pout like a child who isn't getting what she wants. She is happy, then violent, and back to happy again."

I watch Kate's face for a reaction, but I can tell she is not getting it. I don't think she believes us. I don't know how to convince her how severe Janni's violence really is.

Janni makes a move toward Susan and Bodhi.

"Janni." I am on her, my hands on her shoulders, ready to take her out of the room.

Instinctively, Susan holds up her hand, ready to defend Bodhi.

But Janni only leans against Susan. "I want to go," she whines, very much like a normal kid.

"We'll go in a minute," Susan tells her.

Janni punches Susan's arm, hard enough that it sounds like a tennis ball bouncing off a hard wall. But again there is no anger. It is like she is doing it to pass the time.

"Janni, stop!" Susan commands.

Janni's face doesn't change, but her body seems to respond on its own, bringing up both fists and alternating punches into Susan.

I jump in and pull Janni off. Janni goes limp in my hands, giving in, as if hitting Susan really wasn't that interesting after all. I turn back to Kate.

"See? This is what we are dealing with, although it is much worse at home."

Kate looks shocked again.

"Janni, how do you think that feels to your mommy? Do you think she likes being hit?"

"Yes," Janni answers, as if she was just asked if she likes vanilla ice cream.

"Has somebody ever hit you?"

"Daddy."

"When did I hit you, Janni?" I demand.

"When I was bad. When I was trying to hit Bodhi."

"I didn't hit you, Janni. I restrained you. I was terrified you might seriously hurt Bodhi. I didn't know what else to do. I don't let anyone hurt you and I can't let anyone hurt him. You are both my children."

"Well, Janni, did you like what your dad did?"

"Not Janni!" Janni yells like she's told this woman her name a thousand times before. "I'm 76!"

Kate recoils again, smoothing her sweater, then repeating the question.

"No," Janni answers.

"Why not?"

"Because it hurt."

Kate leans forward in her chair. "What you are doing to your mother right now is hurting her. Do you realize that?"

"Yes. I want to hurt her," Janni replies.

Kate's mouth falls open. She clearly wasn't expecting Janni's answer. She regathers her composure and asks, "Why?"

"I want to go," Janni whines.

"Anything else?" the therapist asks.

"No."

Janni hits Susan again.

Bodhi wakes up and starts to cry.

"Bodhi! Be quiet!" Janni screams at him.

This, as expected, makes Bodhi cry harder.

Janni screams and Bodhi erupts into a full-blown wail.

Janni moves to kick his car seat. I grab her and pull her back.

"I've got to get her out of here," I say.

As I am struggling with Janni, Kate swivels to her desk and retrieves a pen and a Post-it note. "I think it might be beneficial for Janni . . ."

"I'm not Janni!" Janni tries to kick out at Kate.

". . . to see a psychiatrist. I know one in Glendale who is really great with kids."

I look sharply back at Kate. "Don't you think she just needs some therapy to work through her emotions?" I ask.

Kate continues writing. "I think therapy might be beneficial in the future, but she needs to be stabilized first. Her name is Dr. Howe,"

Kate continues. "I have referred kids to her before. Usually it takes a while to get an appointment, but I will call her and let her know there's an infant in the home and it's an emergency."

An emergency? This hits me like a brick. Yes, I think Janni's behavior needs immediate attention, but hearing those words from a child psychologist with thirty years of experience terrifies me.

CHAPTER SEVEN

New Year's Eve, 2007

D r. Howe at least has toys in her office. There is a dollhouse and Janni is playing with it.

"Do you like dolls?" Dr. Howe asks.

Janni holds up a six-inch man. "This is 47."

"He's forty-seven?"

"No, his name is 47." Janni picks up the mother doll. "This is 48."

"And what about the baby?" Howe asks.

"50."

"You like numbers?"

Susan pipes in. "She tested with a 146 IQ. I have her IQ test here." She gets out a copy and holds it toward Dr. Howe.

"I don't need to see that," Dr. Howe replies, not taking her eyes off Janni. "I can already tell she is very intelligent."

I'm relieved, still clinging to the belief that the source of Janni's violence is a disconnect between the age of her body and the age of her mind.

Janni gets up and holds out an empty palm to Dr. Howe. "This is my rat, Wednesday."

"I see. What kind of rat is Wednesday?"

"Black-and-white."

"I see. Is Wednesday really there?"

"Yes," Janni answers, then returns her attention to the dolls. She is not playing with them, just naming them.

"Janni, do you know why you're here?" Dr. Howe asks.

"I hit Bodhi," she answers flatly.

I jump in. "She's never actually hit him. We're always there to protect him."

"Okay." Dr. Howe nods and turns back to Janni. "Can you control that?"

"Sometimes I can and sometimes I can't," Janni responds.

Dr. Howe spins her chair around to face us. "I believe her."

She turns her chair to Janni. "Janni, can you keep playing while I talk with your mom and dad?"

"Yeah," Janni agrees, still focused on the dolls.

Dr. Howe turns to us. "So what's been going on?"

Susan starts to talk about the endless violent explosions. Dr. Howe listens and then asks us about our family histories.

"I was on Ritalin from five years old to thirteen," I answer.

Susan chimes in with "And then there was my grandmother's brother, who spent his whole life in Napa State Hospital. He had schizophrenia. My dad said he used to scream all the time." She pauses for a moment, a look of fear coming over her face. "Could she have schizophrenia?"

Schizophrenia? I think to myself, looking at Susan like she's crazy. I don't know what this is, but it sure as hell isn't schizophrenia.

Schizophrenia is the worst mental illness known to mankind. Schizophrenics are those people raving to themselves on street corners.

"We don't want to go there," Dr. Howe states forcefully.

"So, have you seen these behaviors before?" Susan asks.

Dr. Howe looks at her notes, bobbing her head, as if trying to decide what she wants to say. "I have seen some of these behaviors before," she looks up at us, "but not in a child as young as Janni."

"I'm not Janni!" Janni screams.

"Oh, I'm sorry," Dr. Howe tells her, respectfully. "I forgot."

"When she had her IQ tested at four, the therapist said then that she was mentally between ten and eleven. That was over a year ago. Maybe she's mentally a teenager now and this is some sort of teenage rebellion," I suggest.

Dr. Howe shakes her head again. "I don't think that is happening here."

"So what is going on?" I press, wanting a damn diagnosis, an explanation for what is happening to Janni, to our family.

"I'm not prepared to make a diagnosis after just one visit," Dr. Howe responds. "To be honest, we may not be able to figure out a diagnosis for a while."

"But we can't go on living like this," Susan cries.

Dr. Howe nods. "I understand. That is why I am going to prescribe Risperdal. We don't need to know what it is in order to treat the symptoms."

"What's Risperdal?" I ask.

"It's an antipsychotic."

"An antipsychotic?" Susan repeats, alarmed.

"Risperdal is also used to treat anxiety. The lowest dose available is a half miligram. I want you to cut that in half."

"So you think this is just anxiety?" Susan asks hopefully.

Dr. Howe, writing up the prescription, shakes her head.

"Like I said, it's still too early to tell."

She hands me the prescription for Risperdal. "Let's see how she does on this, and we'll make another appointment for her in two weeks."

I stare at the prescription in my hand. Risperdal. An antipsychotic. But I am so tired of living in fear I will try anything.

CHAPTER EIGHT

New Year's Day, 2008

We pull into a local park. The weather is cold, spitting rain. Across the muddy, puddle-filled soccer field from the parking lot the playground is empty. Of course it is. Only the insane would be out on a day like this. I brought Janni out to give Bodhi a few hours of peace. With Janni gone, now he can cry and be safe. It's practically a necessity now to keep Janni away from Bodhi as much as possible. Here I can play with her like I used to.

As Janni gets out of the car I check the clock on the dash.

"Wait, Janni," I say, reaching for the pill bottle. "You've got to take your next dosage."

She stops outside the car, door still open, and looks back at me.

"Risperdal?" she asks.

I nod. She's only five but knows exactly what and how much she's supposed to take.

I open the pill bottle and all I see are full tablets. Dammit. I cut the previous night's dose with a butter knife but forgot to cut more. I don't have a pill cutter, so I put the pill between my teeth and bite down, feeling the spray of powder in my mouth as the back half of the tablet shatters. Shit. I was trying for two complete halves so I could spit the other half into the bottle for later.

I hand the complete half to Janni, along with a bottle of water. She takes it and swallows it.

I turn my head and try to spit out the fragments of Risperdal in my mouth, but they're too small. The chalky sensation is driving me crazy, so I grab a bottle of water and take a swig, swallowing the remainder of the pill.

Janni is waiting in the rain by the open passenger door.

"Let's go," she whines.

"You go on ahead. I'll be right there."

Janni runs off across the muddy soccer field. I watch her go. There is nobody around, so I don't have to worry about anyone grabbing her. Not that I worry about that anyway. After having been on the receiving end of Janni's violence several times, I have no doubt Janni can defend herself from any predator.

I call my dad on my cell phone.

"Hellooo," he bellows. "Happy New Year!"

I'd actually forgotten it was New Year's Day. Normally, Susan would be filling in today for one of the full-time traffic reporters, making double time since it's a holiday, but not this year. It's simply too dangerous for either of us to take both kids.

"Yeah, you, too."

"Do you have anything special planned?" he asks.

I realize we haven't spoken since he left the day after Bodhi was born. It feels like forever, but it's only been two weeks. I fill him in.

Silence. "Dad, are you still there?"

"Yeah, Mike. I just can't believe it, that's all. Jesus Christ."

"Dr. Howe put Janni on a drug called Risperdal. It's an anti-psychotic."

"Jesus Christ," he repeats, still in shock. "Is . . . is this, whatever this drug is called, working?"

I look out through the rain-streaked windshield at Janni, who is swinging by herself.

"I don't know. I don't think so. She still tries to go after Bodhi."

"Well, Mike, do whatever you have to so you keep her away from him until this gets figured out."

Something about his tone angers me. It's like he's giving up on Janni.

"Dad, she is a good kid. She just needs help."

"I understand that, but your primary responsibility has to be to keep Bodhi safe. He can't defend himself."

"I know that. Anyway, the reason I was calling is because Dr. Howe wanted me to ask you if we have any history of mental illness in our family."

"Not that I'm aware of."

I suck in my breath. "What about my mother?"

There's silence on the other end. Dad hates it whenever I bring up my mother. He would prefer the past be left in the past.

"What about her?" he finally says. "Your mother was never diagnosed with anything to my knowledge."

"I know that, but clearly there was something wrong with her."

"Well, I won't dispute that."

"Do you think she had a mental illness?"

"Shit, Mike, I don't know."

"She believed you were a hit man for the Mafia, Dad, and that you had a million dollars stashed away in a Singapore bank."

"Well, she certainly had some strange ideas, but I can't say whether she was mentally ill or what kind of mental illness she might have had."

"Is there anyone else in our family you can think of?"

"Not off the top of my head. Nothing like what you're describing."

"Wasn't there someone in our family who committed suicide?" I ask, annoyed. Getting my father to talk about our past is like pulling teeth.

"My cousin," Dad replies. "Peg's son." Peg is my great-aunt and our last surviving relative from Australia, where I was born. "He hung himself."

"How old was he?"

"In his fifties."

"Was he ever diagnosed with anything?"

"Schizophrenia," Dad answers.

I let the word hang there for a moment. Not what I wanted to hear.

"So there was someone in our family with schizophrenia," I say.

"Well, I don't know that he really had it."

"What do you mean?"

"He got the diagnosis after he was arrested for stealing a car. I think he probably convinced them he was schizophrenic to avoid going to jail."

"That doesn't mean he didn't have it."

"I spent a lot of time with him when we were growing up. He came down to Sydney back in the sixties, supposedly to find a job, which he never did. I talked to him a lot, and he only ever brought up being schizophrenic when he got into some kind of trouble with the law. He just didn't want to work. Basically, Michael, he was a bum. Honestly, I think he finally killed himself because life was too hard."

That is what I am afraid of. Life is hard for Janni, too.

I hang up the phone and get out of the car when I see Janni starting to wander around the park, obviously bored. I have to get over there and keep her engaged. I have nowhere else to go with her, and I sure as hell won't take her home yet.

I step onto the soccer field and instantly my feet disappear under a thin layer of muddy water. I didn't realize it was this deep. Water is running over the tops of my shoes and soaking my feet. I start to lift my opposing foot to walk forward, but the mud grabs at my feet.

Janni looks over and sees me coming. "Daddy, come play with me!"

Walking through the mud is very difficult. My steps are getting more deliberate.

"Daddy, come on!" Janni is getting impatient.

"I'm coming!" I call, still plodding. This is hard, tiring work. I realize I am breathing heavily from the effort. I stop for a moment to catch my breath.

"Daddy, are you coming?"

Of course I'm coming. I glance back at the car in shock. I've only gone about fifty feet. Janni is still more than a hundred feet away.

I take another step, then another. It takes everything I have to pull my feet free of the mud and move them forward.

I stop again, needing to rest. I look up at Janni and it is like I haven't moved at all. Every few steps, I have to catch my breath. It dawns on me that something is wrong.

You just swallowed half of a Risperdal tablet, I remember.

No, I think, dismissing the thought. This can't possibly be the Risperdal. I only swallowed a little bit and that was just a few minutes ago. It can't possibly have kicked in yet.

"Daddy!" Janni calls. "I want you to come play with me."

I lift my leg and then realize I am too tired to take another step. I have an intense urge to just lie down and go to sleep.

Janni watches me. Even from here I can see the look of concern on her face. "Daddy? Are you okay?"

I manage one more step and the effort wipes me out. *This can't possibly be the Risperdal. It's a kid's dosage and I'm five times her weight, yet Janni took the same dose and she's fine.*

"I'll be right there, sweetie," I call. "Just go back to playing and I'll be right there."

"But I want you," she whines.

"I'll be right there," I yell. It is all I can do to keep standing up.

Janni sullenly turns away.

"Fine. I'll play with 24 Hours instead." 24 Hours is a girl, the first human imaginary friend Janni has created. Janni has no human friends anymore. She runs off through the playground, climbing the equipment, yelling out to 24 Hours. I look down at my own body, which suddenly feels hundreds of pounds heavier, then up at Janni. This is impossible. I know one of Risperadal's side effects is sedation, yet it hasn't had any sedative effect on Janni. She is still running around. No one would know she's on any medication at all.

CHAPTER NINE

January 2008

I have to teach at 8 A.M., so I'm speeding, weaving in between slower cars, when Bodhi starts crying in the back. I know my driving is scaring him, but I don't have a choice. I'll still be late to CSUN, and the class is only fifty minutes long.

I'm driving Bodhi to Susan's old roommate, Jeanne, which I do every weekday morning now. I was offered these classes last September, three months before Bodhi was born, and I took them without hesitation. I only graduated with my MA nine months ago and already I get enough classes at CSUN that I don't need to be one of the "freeway flyers," part-time college instructors who have to shuttle from college to college to pick up enough classes to pay the bills. Taking these early-morning classes the more senior instructors don't want is how I've achieved that. But that was before Janni became violent.

Susan and I both wake up before dawn. While I shower and shave, she gets Bodhi dressed and packs his diaper bag. This way when

Janni wakes up in the morning, Bodhi won't be there and Susan won't have to lock the door, keeping Bodhi inside with her, while she takes a shower.

I pull into the driveway of Jeanne's house. Leaving the car running, I detach Bodhi's car seat from its holder and carry him to the front door. I put him down on the front stoop, ring the bell, and race back to the car to retrieve his stroller.

Jeanne opens the front door, still in her nightgown. "Hi, little man," she coos, bending down to pick Bodhi up out of his car seat. I stand in the driveway with the stroller, watching them. I'm glad Susan doesn't have to see Bodhi leaning against Jeanne like she is his mother.

She turns to me. "Hi, Michael."

"Open the trunk of your car so I can put his stroller in the back" is my response. In the back of my mind, I know I am being brusque, rude even, but I don't want to talk. I don't want to think. If I think, I will have to deal with feelings I don't have time for right now.

Jeanne goes into her house to retrieve her car keys. "How are things? How is Janni?"

"The same," I answer quickly, unlocking her trunk and loading in Bodhi's stroller.

"Doesn't the doctor have any ideas?" she asks, bouncing Bodhi up and down in her arms.

"She wants Janni to see a neurologist," I answer, "to rule out any brain damage. Because so far the antipsychotics aren't working."

"I can't believe she is on antipsychotics," Jeanne replies, shaking her head in dismay.

I slam the trunk closed. "Are you okay for diapers?"

"Uh, I think so."

"Okay, I'll be back to pick him up at twelve-thirty." I get back in the car and back out of the driveway.

I floor the accelerator, racing down the street, away from my six-week-old son. I didn't say or kiss good-bye to Bodhi. I never do. I can't even bring myself to look at him when I leave, because I am afraid if I do, if I see his eyes meet mine, I will collapse into a blubbering mess. Jeanne has a daughter, too, Lauren, who's a year younger than Janni. Every time I return to get Bodhi, Lauren is sitting over Bodhi, talking to him, playing with him, and making him laugh. I'd never heard him laugh until I brought him here. I watch them together and it hurts. Lauren is like the big sister Janni was supposed to be.

THE EEG TECH puts the first conductor on Janni's forehead and she immediately pulls it off.

"Janni, you have to leave that on," I order her.

"It's cold," she complains.

"That's just the gel they put on to increase the conductivity of the electrical activity in your brain. I know it's cold, but it will warm up to your body temperature very quickly."

"I won't do it," Janni replies.

"Janni, don't you want to see what your brain waves look like? It will be like seeing your own thoughts!"

"No." Janni gets up out of her chair and moves for the door.

I grab her.

"If she is not going to be able to do this today," the tech says, holding dozens of electrical wires in her hand, "we could reschedule to a day where she's in a better mood."

"This is always her mood," I say irritably, thinking, *Why the hell do you think we are here?* "There isn't going to be a better day."

"In order to get an accurate reading," the tech replies, "I need her to sit perfectly still. Even the slightest movement can affect the readout."

"For how long?" I ask.

"Ideally, about thirty minutes."

I exhale, frustrated.

"There is no way she's going to sit still for thirty minutes." I had hoped this dumb woman would help me by engaging Janni, teaching her about the EEG machine and what she is doing, but she's not making any effort at all. I have no patience anymore for anyone who can't help me with Janni.

"If you don't think she can do it awake, we can put her under anesthesia."

"Can we do that now?" I ask hopefully.

The tech shakes her head. "No. That would have to be done at a hospital."

"Janni, do you want to go to the hospital?" Susan asks, making me jump. I'd actually forgotten she was here. Not that it makes any difference. It might as well just be me. I am the only one who can get Janni through this. I'll teach her, be silly, do whatever I have to do.

"No," Janni answers.

"Then come on," I urge her. "Let's get through this."

It takes twenty minutes just to get the electrodes on Janni's head. She keeps complaining they are cold and trying to take them off, but I hold both her hands in mine and keep talking to her, trying to teach her about EEG machines and brain waves.

Finally, every electrode is on.

"See, Janni? I told you it doesn't hurt."

"I want them off!"

"Just keep focused on me," I tell her. "Focus on my eyes."

"Okay," the tech says. "Try to hold perfectly still."

Janni shifts in the chair and, pulling one of her hands free from mine, reaches up for the wires going into her head.

I quickly grab hold of her hands to prevent her from pulling off the electrodes.

"Are you getting it?" I ask the tech, not taking my eyes of Janni.

"She needs to not move," the tech replies.

"Janni, just hold still, okay?"

"I want to get out!" she cries, trying to twist free of me.

I feel for her. Even a normal kid would have a hard time sitting for an EEG, let alone Janni. But we need answers, some explanation for her violence.

"Just hold on, Janni," I repeat calmly. "Do you want to see what your brain waves look like?"

Janni nods.

"She can't move her head," the tech says sharply.

"If she can see them she might stay still," I reply, increasingly pissed off with this tech.

Janni turns her head to see the readout, allowing me to look, too. There are eight lines, all moving at different speeds.

"Those are your brain waves," I say to Janni.

Janni turns back, which frustrates me. I would have expected her to be fascinated by this. Every time she moves, several of the lines on the screen jump wildly.

"I want to go," Janni says again. "Please get me out of this."

I sigh, losing hope. "Are you able to get anything?" I ask the tech.

"Let me go ask the doctor and see what he wants to do." The tech leaves.

While she's gone, in between trying to keep Janni from pulling her electrodes out, I watch the screen, trying to see if I can identify something unusual, like one wave jumping wildly. But they are all pretty much the same.

The tech comes back. "The doctor said it would be nice to get thirty minutes, but we don't need it. If she can just sit still for two minutes, that will be enough to get her baseline."

Hope rises again. "Did you hear that, Janni? Just two minutes. You can do two minutes."

I count down from one hundred and twenty. When Janni moves after ninety seconds, I want to scream. We were so close!

"Janni! We only had thirty seconds to go!"

"I want to get out!" she cries.

The tech starts to remove the electrodes. "We're done," she says.

I slump, dejected. "So we're going to have to do the hospital."

The tech shakes her head. "No, I think we've got enough to at least get a sense if there's anything abormal."

"Is there?" Susan asks, again reminding me she's actually here.

"The doctor needs to analyze the printout."

"Can he do that today?" I ask.

"He can't today."

I am so frustrated. I want to know. No, I need to know. I don't know how many more times I can take holding Janni down during one of her rages, looking into her eyes, and seeing something else other than my daughter. I need to know what that "something else" is. Then I need to know how to stop it.

TWO WEEKS LATER we go back to the neurologist to get the results of the EEG.

Everything is normal.

I can't believe it. I am so desperate for answers that I would actually have been relieved if I'd been told she had a tumor. I will accept any explanation for the violence. But still no one has one.

"Janni wasn't able to sit still for very long. Are you sure you got enough?" I ask, prepared to do it again, putting Janni under general anesthetic this time.

The neurologist shakes his head. "We got what we needed. The point was to look for anything abnormal, and there isn't anything."

I am devastated. We're back to square one.

"So do you have any idea what is causing her behavior?" I ask weakly.

"You need to go back and talk to Dr. Howe," he replies. "We've ruled out physical causes. It's not for me to say anything else."

I persist. "Consider it a second opinion."

The neurologist watches Janni bounce around his office, unable to sit still, picking up things and throwing them. "Honestly, I think it's ADHD."

ADHD? That's supposedly what I had. Why I was on the Ritalin.

I'd always believed that I didn't need it, that I was given it simply because my mother couldn't handle me. But I'm not so sure anymore. I take Lexapro, which is an antidepressant. I've tried different antidepressants for years, but none of them worked until Lexapro. Maybe that was because my depression didn't manifest as sadness.

I got angry . . . just like Janni.

CHAPTER TEN

Early February 2008

We're on our way to Pump It Up, an indoor play area in Woodland Hills, a half-hour drive away and a good test to see if Janni and Bodhi can ride in the same car while she's on her new Ritalin medication.

As usual, as soon as we start driving, Bodhi starts crying, but this time, Janni doesn't react. It's like she doesn't hear him crying. We still have her in the front passenger seat next to me, while Susan rides in the back next to Bodhi.

When we get to the play area, I am shocked to see only babies and toddlers.

"Where are the kids Janni's age?" I ask Susan.

Susan is settling down with Bodhi, preparing to feed him.

"It's a school day," she replies.

I feel a pang of pain in my heart. I'd forgotten that Janni should be in school by now. Janni's peers are growing up, while Janni appears to be stuck. The world is moving on without her, I think sadly, remembering my image of her as a shut-in.

I don't expect Janni to last long at the play area. I figure if we get an hour we will be doing well. To my shock, Janni starts helping the younger kids climb into the tunnels or into the ball pit. *She's interacting with other kids!*

The Ritalin is the answer to our prayers, a miracle drug. Not only is her violence gone, but here she is, busy helping the younger children. I haven't seen her be nice to another child since she was a toddler herself, and now here she is, holding their hands, taking them back to their mothers when they get scared, reassuring them. She is suddenly the big sister I always hoped she would be.

Every so often she runs back to us, but instead of talking about her imaginary friends, she talks about the other children, giving us their names and how old they are.

She is talking a mile a minute. She has always been a fast talker, but this is even faster.

I have read up on Ritalin, just as I have on Risperdal. Like all ADHD drugs, it's supposed to calm a child down. The fact that it is winding Janni up can mean only one thing: Janni doesn't have ADHD.

"She's very wound up," I say to Susan after Janni runs back to play with the toddlers. "It's like she's high."

"But at least she's not being violent," Susan replies. "I would rather her be high and happy than unhappy and violent."

I agree. So Ritalin makes our daughter high as a kite. At least she's happy and the violence is gone.

AFTER A FULL day of playing at Pump It Up, we get into the car and drive home. I start to think my original belief was correct: The source of Janni's rage is a disconnect between her brilliant mind and her young body. It's been making her depressed, and that makes her become violent. The Ritalin makes her high, thereby taking away the violence.

It is early evening and traffic is heavy. Bodhi starts to cry. Given that she didn't scream at him when he cried on the drive here, I am taken by surprise when Janni suddenly screams at him to be quiet.

Okay, I tell myself. *Don't panic. The Ritalin is just wearing off.* I tell Susan to give her another pill.

"But if I give her one now, she won't sleep," Susan protests. "We're only supposed to give it to her in the morning."

Janni takes off her shoes and unbuckles her seat belt, turning around to throw her shoes at Bodhi. I grab at her arms, my eyes going back and forth between the road in front of me and Janni.

"If you don't give her one now," I roar, "we'll never make it home."

Janni keeps screaming at Bodhi and trying to hit him, while Susan searches in her purse for the bottle of Ritalin.

"Janni, put on the headphones." I reach down to the floor of the passenger side and retrieve the headphones I bought for Janni. They're designed for shooters, rated to block out thirty-five decibels. I've tried them on myself, and I know they won't completely eliminate the sound of Bodhi's crying, but they do dull the sound so it's like he's yards away.

I slip them over Janni's head, but she rips them off, slamming her hands over her ears.

"Janni, I told you to wear the headphones!"

"I can still hear him!" she wails.

"But they will dull his crying," I insist.

"They don't! I can still hear him!"

"But not as loud."

Janni violently shakes her head. "It's still the same!"

I don't get this. How can it be the same? It's almost like the sound of Bodhi's crying is inside her head.

. . .

A FEW HOURS later it's nighttime.

"Her eyes are dilated and her heart is beating faster than ever," Susan shouts to me from her bedroom. I'm on the couch by Bodhi, zoning out on TV.

"You should go to bed," I tell Susan. "I'll stay up with her until she goes to sleep. You wanna watch *Survivorman*?"

"Yes," Janni answers, and she snuggles beside me on the couch. This is one of our favorite shows.

Susan and I make eye contact. "No more Ritalin," she says.

I nod. Another medication we can't rely on. The second dose never kicked in. I drove all the way home, with my arm guarding Janni, while Susan shielded the screaming Bodhi with her body. It took us two hours to get home because of traffic. And now she can't fall asleep. Her heart is racing.

I put my hand on Janni's chest. It's still fast. From the moment it first begins to beat, the heart has an internal clock. Genetics has programmed a certain number of beats, and when that number is up, the heart will stop. The faster it goes, the closer to the end we get.

I am terrified.

CHAPTER ELEVEN

Valentine's Day, 2008

I t feels strange to be standing outside a public school, waiting for Janni to finish afternoon kindergarten. For so long we thought we'd be homeschooling Janni. Because of her high IQ, we knew she would be bored out of her mind with public school, but there is no way she would pass the entrance interview for Mirman and I have to work. Janni is still a danger to Bodhi, so we have no choice but to put her somewhere and this is our only option.

"How was school?" Susan asks nervously as Janni comes out to greet us. We're both on eggshells hoping today was better than yesterday, or any of the days since she started.

"Fine," Janni answers.

"Janni," the kindergarten teacher calls. "Don't forget your backpack."

Janni runs to get her backpack and brings it over to where we are standing. She pulls out her red folder and removes a heart cut from red construction paper. "I made this for you." She hands it to me, excited. I read it: "HAPPY VALENTINE'S DAY, FROM 76."

"Thank you, Janni, I love it."

Janni smiles and runs off to the playground. Susan tells her that one of the girls from her class is at the playground, too. I watch, always hoping to see Janni playing with another child. But she never even looks at her classmate.

"Do you have a minute?" the teacher calls to us.

"You go in today," Susan says under her breath to me. "I'm tired of talking to them. They don't get it and I'm tired of explaining."

Susan wheels Bodhi's stroller after Janni while I head for the classroom. I already know this is going to be about Janni's behavior. It is always about Janni's behavior.

As I walk, I look at the other papers inside the red folder. On top is a small piece of white paper, Janni's behavioral report for the day: *Didn't want to participate in activities. Screamed. Hit another child.*

I look underneath at her work for the day. Every sheet is either scribbled all over or ripped in two, both things Janni will do if she makes a mistake. Rather than just taking an eraser and erasing it like she's supposed to, she acts like the mistake is written in stone. Some of the torn sheets are completely blank. When I look at the top of the sheet, I see why. The teacher wrote "January," which will automatically make Janni tear it up.

"So how did she do?" I ask, stupidly, hoping for some good news.

The teacher, a nice enough young woman, fresh out of college, shrugs. "She had to go to the principal's office for a while because she wouldn't stop hitting."

My daughter is five and already being sent to the principal's office. She knows him by name, something I am certain no other child in her class does.

"I also really need her to write her name," she adds.

"Yeah, I know. She doesn't like her name," I reply.

"But one of the requirements of kindergarten is that students be able to write their first names by the time the school year is done. She needs to do it. It is a California requirement."

This isn't unreasonable, but it still pisses me off. She has a 146 IQ, but they don't give a damn about that. All that matters to them is the stupid rules.

"What about teaching her science?" I ask.

"I do. In fact, when it's just Janni and me, she's wonderful. It's only when I have to move on to help another student that things get rough. It's like if I could be with her all the time, she would be perfect."

I look over at the whiteboard. Every student's name is up there in one of three columns: green, yellow, and red. The teacher calls it the "Streetlight System." Names written in green are the students who are following directions, green meant to indicate that they can "go," or continue as they are doing. Names in yellow are students who have been asked to "slow down" and think about what they are doing. Names in red are students who have been told to stop. Janni's name is always either in yellow or red. I have never seen her name in green.

"Red again," I comment.

The teacher is sympathetic. "The system works well for other students but not for Janni. She doesn't care. That is why I had to send her to the principal's office. That's the next step if a 'red light' is ignored."

I hate putting Janni through this. I know this isn't where she needs to be. The other kids are learning their ABCs and Janni knows the periodic table of elements. I look down at the floor, wishing we could just solve the violence. If we could fix that, then we could home-school her.

CHAPTER TWELVE

Saturday, March 8, 2008

Even though today is Saturday, I am working. I signed up to grade the writing exam every CSUN student must pass in order to graduate. I get $250 for six hours of work, money we desperately need. College lecturers don't make much.

I thought about not doing it because it means Susan has to take both Janni and Bodhi, but she already hired a babysitter for the day, a young college girl named Shawna who manages the toy store in the mall, the same store Janni destroyed two years ago. She saw Janni tear through the store for about a year but seemed to genuinely like her, even engaging her in conversation when she ran behind her cash register. Susan said she has experience as a nanny and works with her autistic nephew, so she understands meltdowns. She is going to help Susan with Janni and Bodhi while I am gone.

I read through the exams, although my mind keeps drifting to what might be happening with Susan and the kids.

By late morning we're given a break and I go out into the corridor and call Susan. "How's it going?"

"Not well," Susan answers, her voice like I've never heard it before. She sounds . . . broken.

"Where are you?"

"Right now I am parked outside the ER at Henry Mayo."

Panic squeezes my blood vessels. "Why are you there? What happened?"

On top of my fears of Janni hurting Bodhi, I now live in constant fear that Susan is going to put Janni in a psychiatric hospital. Dr. Howe keeps pushing for it because Janni is not responding to medication. Susan agrees, but I can't accept Janni going into a hospital. If we put her in one, I feel like we will have crossed a point of no return. As long as Janni is out of the hospital, there is still hope that, just maybe, this is a phase that she will outgrow.

"She tried to hit Bodhi." Susan starts to cry. "I was driving. She would have done it if Shawna hadn't been here to stop her."

I look down at the floor, angry, not sure what to do. "She always tries to hit him. That doesn't mean you go to the ER."

"It scared Shawna enough that she told me to call 911."

"That's just because she's never seen it before," I reply. "She's not used to it."

"I called 911."

My razor-thin sense of control is beginning to crack.

"Why?!" I whine.

"Because even Shawna couldn't control her! I didn't know what else to do. They just told me to take her to the emergency room. By the time I got here, she was asleep."

I exhale, relieved. *An ambulance didn't come. They didn't take Janni away.*

"Hold on," I say. "I'm on my way."

"She's asleep right now. When she wakes up, she is still going to want to do something. Just meet me at the party."

AFTER I'M DONE grading the exams, I race to the birthday party at Color Me Mine in Porter Ranch. It's midway between where I work in Northridge and where we live in Valencia.

When I get inside, I see Susan, standing, holding Bodhi, talking to the mother of the girl whose birthday it is.

"Where's Janni?" I demand.

Susan looks around. "I'm not sure."

I leave her, ignoring Bodhi, who was the victim, searching for Janni. I find her sitting at one of the tables, painting a ceramic dog. Half the dog's head is purple and the other half is yellow, the purple bleeding over into the lighter color.

There is plenty of room to sit down next to her, because there are no kids anywhere close.

"How're you doing?" I ask her, like nothing bad has happened.

"Fine," she answers.

I look around at the other girls. They are painting, too, but it is different. They paint and chatter among themselves. I look back at Janni, who gives no indication that she is aware of anybody else.

One of the staff comes over and picks up the dog. "What's your name, sweetie?" she asks. "I need to write on the bottom so we know who this belongs to."

"Eloise," Janni answers.

The woman looks at me. "Eloise? Like in the books?"

"Yes," I answer. "We're big fans." I am not going to give Janni's real name. I am not going to trigger her. Besides, I'm pretty confident that there are no other "Eloises" at this party.

"I want to go," Janni says without looking at me. But she isn't

76

whining. She is begging, as if being here, surrounded by all these other children, is causing her physical pain.

"Okay," I answer, getting up immediately. I want to get her out of here. I want to get her away from any place and any person that reminds her she is different. Or reminds me.

Susan is still talking to the other mothers. I say nothing as we leave, angry that she keeps putting Janni in situations like this.

WE ARE DRIVING. I don't know where, exactly. I just want to get Janni away.

"Mommy thinks I need to go to the hospital," Janni says quietly.

My first instinct is to say, *Your mother is full of shit,* but I don't. Susan is still her mother. "Do you feel you need to go?" I ask her instead.

"I don't want to go to the hospital, but I think I need to."

This hits me like a sledgehammer.

"Why?" I ask, almost choking on the words.

"I want to hit Bodhi all the time. I can't help it."

My five-year-old daughter is telling me she thinks she needs to be hospitalized. It is more than I can bear, so in that moment I get angry with Susan again. If Susan had a full-time job, I could stay with Janni all the time. She just can't fit into our world, our system, our rules. If I could take her, I could protect her from society. I want to keep driving, just her and me, into the desert, as far away as I can get.

"It'll be okay, Janni," I tell her. "We'll get through this."

CHAPTER THIRTEEN

Sunday, March 9, 2008

Our dog Honey, an Australian shepherd–golden retriever mix, hasn't been able to run in weeks, and since Susan wanted to spend some time with Janni alone, here I am with Bodhi, his body propped against me, his head on my shoulder.

He's not even three months. He snuggles into me, seemingly just happy to be held. Janni was never like this. Even at this age, she was always struggling, trying to get down, wanting to move, to explore. Bodhi is nice to hold. I give him a kiss on the side of his head.

My cell phone rings and I retrieve it from my pocket. I don't bother to check caller ID anymore. It's always Susan.

"Are you at the Pizza Kitchen yet?"

I expect Susan to tell me Janni is doing fine on their "girls' day out."

"We're at Alhambra," Susan answers flatly.

"What?" BHC Alhambra is a psychiatric hospital. I look around for Honey, wanting to get her back on the leash and get out of here. Maybe they are still en route. Maybe I can still stop this.

"Just come back and I will take Janni," I say, trying to control my anger.

"It's too late. They've already taken her back." Susan sounds spent but relieved.

I turn in circles, trying to spot Honey, feeling powerless. "Why?" It's a rhetorical question. I know why, but I still can't accept it.

"She was hitting me and throwing things at me nonstop. I just couldn't take it anymore."

"Why didn't you call me?!"

"Because she needed to go. You even told me last night that she said she needed to go."

I spot Honey and scream at her to come.

"Don't yell at Honey," Susan tells me. "Let her have her time."

Susan just checked our five-year-old daughter into a psych ward and she's upset that I am yelling at Honey?

"I tried!" I hear Susan say. "I really did! I thought we could work through it."

I am furious. I never should have let Susan take her. I should have known she couldn't handle Janni, even without Bodhi.

"You should have called me before you took her," I hiss.

"She wants to go. She needs help, help we can't provide."

"You mean you can't provide," I answer bitterly. I feel like Susan has taken my child from me.

I HAVE TO take Honey home before I go to Alhambra, more than forty miles from where we live.

I put Bodhi's car seat down on the floor of Janni's bedroom.

Susan wants me to pack a bag of clothes for Janni, so I get her

Disney Princess suitcase out of the closet and lay it down on the carpet next to Bodhi. I slip down to the carpet next to the suitcase and stare at it. On the bed in front of me is Hero, Janni's favorite bear. I stand and pick up Hero. I don't want to pack clothes for Janni. If I pack clothes, then that means she is staying. I wonder if I have the guts to go there and pull her out. Would Susan fight me on that? I don't know. I don't know if I can trust her anymore. She is clearly cracking under the stress.

I sigh and put Hero into the bag. I will pack clothes. But if when I get there Janni is scared and wants to leave, I am going to take her, whether Susan likes it or not.

WHEN I FINALLY find BHC Alhambra and pull into the parking lot, it is nothing like what I expected. It doesn't look like a hospital at all. I get out of the car and stare at the twelve-foot-high steel bars that surround what appears to be an outside patio area. The final twelve inches at the top of the bars curve inward. I know what this is for. Down the highway from us is our local water reservoir. It is also surrounded by a security perimeter with a fence where the final foot curves. Such a curve makes it impossible to climb over the fence. The direction of the curve tells you whether the fence is designed to keep people in or out. At the reservoir, the fence curves out toward the freeway. Here at Alhambra, the top of the fence curves in, toward the hospital, to stop people from getting out.

Okay, I say to myself, *I get that.* This is a psychiatric facility. Most people who are brought to a place like this are brought here against their will. When I was sixteen, I spent two weeks as a patient in a psychiatric ward for troubled kids. My father didn't give me a choice. My parents had divorced and I went to live with my father, but after what I'd been through with my mother, I couldn't adapt to a "normal" life again. I started doing drugs. I ran away from home. I set fires. Eventually, my father told me that if I wanted to live with him I had to go to a place where

I would get the help I needed. I remember there were bars on the windows of that place as well. But the place I was in was on the fifth floor of a full hospital. There were appendectomies below and babies being born above me. This place is just one floor. There is no ER, no signs to surgery or maternity. This is not a full hospital. It's more like a prison. Janni is only a five-year-old child. She shouldn't be in a place like this.

Susan is sitting in the waiting room, bent over a clipboard, when I enter, pushing Bodhi's stroller and pulling Janni's bag.

"Oh, good, you're here," she says, as if I just got home. She puts the clipboard down. "You can finish the rest of this. I've been filling out paperwork for two hours."

I can't believe how Susan is acting. She looks relaxed.

I appear calm, but it is taking all my effort not to run back into the facility and save Janni. It's been years, but I still remember looking down from the window of my room in the psych ward, watching my father's car drive away. I cried myself to sleep that night.

"Where is she?"

"She's back on the kids' unit," Susan replies, gesturing deeper into the building. "We'll be able to go back and see her in a few minutes. It's almost visiting hours. Which are six to seven, by the way."

There are visiting hours? I think to myself. *This is my child and I can only see her for one hour a day?* Forget this. I am not going to let someone tell me when I can or cannot see my child.

"Is she here under a voluntary or does she have a hold?" I ask, remembering the terminology from my own experience. A "hold" means that you can't leave, that a doctor has determined you are a danger to yourself or others. "Voluntary" means you or your parents, if you are a minor, checked you in. I was a voluntary, in the loosest sense of the word, as I was a minor and my father had checked me in.

"It's voluntary, I think," Susan replies, then thinks for a moment. "I had to sign a document giving them permission to treat her. They weren't going to take her at first. The receptionist kept saying there were no beds available, but I told them I wasn't leaving. Eventually, some guy from admissions came out and he started telling me the same thing, that they have no beds. So I just said 'January' to her and of course she blew up and started screaming and hitting me. The admissions guy looked shocked. I kept calling her 'January' and she kept hitting me until the admissions guy took her back. So much for not having any beds, huh?"

I stare at Susan, feeling my anger escalating.

"So you provoked her to get her in here," I say, an edge in my voice.

"I had no choice. Even Dr. Howe says she needs to be here so they can observe her and figure out what is going on. It wasn't easy for me, either. I didn't know if I was making the right choice until we went onto the unit. There's an eight- or nine-year-old boy back there and he told me, 'She has what I have.' That made me feel much better."

It doesn't make me feel any better at all.

When six o'clock rolls around, we head down a long corridor. Susan is pushing Bodhi's stroller. I want to see my daughter. The corridor ends at a door, and I reach for the handle and pull. Nothing happens, so I start yanking on the door like it is stuck.

"We have to wait for the receptionist to open it," Susan tells me.

Of course, I realize, feeling stupid. The door has an electronic lock that must be disengaged from a remote station.

I pull on the door again. Still nothing. I am locked out from my little girl. I would rather deal with the violence and constant fear of her hurting Bodhi. This is much worse. I had the situation under control. All I had to do was keep Janni and Bodhi separated. Now I have no control at all.

"It's still locked," I snap at Susan. "Go tell the receptionist we are locked out."

"You can call on that phone right there," Susan replies, pointing to a phone next to the door.

Once the door finally opens, I find myself in a cafeteria. It looks decent enough, like a cafeteria in any hospital. I see several patients, all adults, eating with family members. I can tell the patients right away, even if I can't see the plastic wristband on their arms that identifies them as such. The patients are all in pajamas, bathrobes, or sweats. Their hair is unkempt, like they haven't bothered to wash it.

I follow Susan as she turns left and exits the cafeteria into a courtyard. We follow a stone path. It looks pleasant enough until we turn another corner and I see a handful of adults sitting outside a building. They are all smoking. I smoke and Janni sees me smoke, but for some reason I don't want Janni exposed to these people. Janni has never been impressionable in her life, has never been able to be influenced, but suddenly I am terrified she will start to identify with these people. What really bothers me is the blank expressions on their faces. I don't know if it is the drugs they're on, or if they've just been beaten down by life, but either way I don't want Janni to start thinking they are what her future will be. Janni is brilliant. Janni is going to go to college as early as she wants to. Janni is going to do something incredible for the human race, like cure cancer. Janni is going to win the Nobel Prize. Janni is not going to bounce in and out of places like this for the rest of her life. I have to get her out of here.

"They have a pool here." Susan points out a fenced-in pool, filled with leaves and sticks, dirty and uninviting. "At least she can go swimming."

I look at Susan like she's nuts. This is not a fucking summer camp. It's a psych ward.

The kids' unit is in the back of the hospital. There's another gate with a phone. Susan tells me I have to pick up the phone and it will automatically ring the nurses' station. As I do, I look up at the twelve-foot-high chain-link fence covering the patio. A giant avocado tree hangs over it. The avocados are rotting, with some having already fallen. I can't take my eyes off the chain-link covering. Why is that even there? Who the hell could climb twelve feet of steel bars? And even if someone could, there is nowhere to go once they got out.

An orderly comes out and unlocks the gate for us. He leads us across the patio and opens the door to the building, gesturing for us to go inside. The first thing that greets me is the cacophony of noise. Above me a TV is blaring *Toy Story*. There are about half a dozen boys sitting in chairs, but none of them are watching the movie. Most of them have shaved heads and matching tan baggy shorts with white T-shirts. In the few seconds it takes us to cross this room, I hear the words "fuck," "shit," and "faggot" several times as they play at beating the crap out of one another, which is what passes for fun in certain neighborhoods of Los Angeles. I can't tell exactly how old any of them are, but all of them seem far older than Janni. I spot one boy, sitting off by himself, hugging his knees and staring straight ahead like he's trying to pretend he is somewhere else. I don't blame him. I would be, too. This is not a psych ward. This is juvenile hall.

"That's the boy who said he knows what Janni has," Susan says, seeing my gaze.

"The girls are through here," the orderly says, inserting his key into the wall next to a set of double doors.

"You keep the boys and girls separate?" I ask, massively relieved.

"During the day," the orderly answers. "At night some of the younger boys come in here to sleep."

They let some of the boys sleep on the same wing as the girls? I think to myself, looking back at the boys. That's it. I am taking Janni out of this place. This is not a hospital. These boys are not here because they have psychological or psychiatric problems. They're probably here because they beat the shit out of someone and are just too young for juvie.

The orderly opens the door and there is Janni. In the middle of the hall, surrounded by girls, none of whom look younger than fifteen.

But she is laughing and clapping her hands excitedly. The girls move as a group for the community room, and Janni goes with them, right in the middle of the pack. Only then does she see me.

"Daddy!" She runs to me, not in fear, but instead like she's having a good time at a sleepover and I have just arrived to pick her up.

"Hey, sweetie." I go down on my knees and take her in my arms, wanting to hold her, wanting to reassure her that Daddy is here now. Daddy is here to save her.

She wriggles free from me.

"Did you bring me Pizza Kitchen?" she asks, smiling, rolling her wrists like she does when she is excited. "Mommy said you were bringing Pizza Kitchen."

I am still trying to take in everything that is happening. Where is the fear?

"Ah, I wanted to get here as quick as I could. Del Taco was on my way, so I got that instead."

Janni frowns and hits me.

"I don't want Del Taco! I want Pizza Kitchen!"

I stare at Janni, not understanding. Who cares about food? Do you realize you're locked up?

"Can you tell me how you are doing?" I ask her, still searching for any signs of fear. *Just say the word, Janni, and I will take you out of here.*

She ignores my question, retrieving the bag of Del Taco from beneath Bodhi's stroller. She goes over to a table, pulls out the French fries, and starts eating.

"Janni, how are you doing?" I ask again. "Are you all right?"

"Fine," she answers, her mouth full. "Just hungry."

This can't be right. "Janni, do you know where you are?" I ask.

"A hospital," she answers as if I'd just asked what two plus two is.

"Do you know why you are here?"

"Because I want to hit Bodhi."

"If you stop trying to hurt Bodhi, you can come home," I remind her.

"I can't stop," she answers.

I am getting increasingly scared. "Do you understand, then, that you are going to have to stay here?"

Janni nods.

"Do you understand that you will be staying here without Mommy or Daddy?" I ask her, convinced she doesn't yet grasp the full extent of what has happened.

She nods again. "I like it here," she says through a mouthful of fries.

No, this is not possible. I wanted to go home. I didn't want to be in a psych ward.

"It's fun," Janni continues.

She seems content. Relaxed.

In a psych ward.

She looks up at me. "Tomorrow can you bring me Pizza Kitchen?"

IT'S FULLY DARK as I drive home. I have the window down, letting the windblast in, so I can chain-smoke, tossing one butt out the window and lighting another immediately after.

Ahead of me I see the taillights of our other car, the one I drove to Alhambra. Susan is driving. Bodhi is asleep in the back.

I can't bear to look at the passenger seat next to me, because it is empty. I left her there. For the first time since Janni came home from the hospital nearly six years ago, she will be going to sleep in a place we are not.

As we were leaving, Susan kept telling me Janni was happy there, like she was trying to reassure herself. "We always wanted to find friends who get her imagination," she said, "and now we have." She paused and started to tear up. "I just never thought we'd find them in a psych ward."

What hurts so much is that I know Susan is right. And that is why I hate her so much right now. Janni was having the time of her life, happier than I can remember her being in years. I wanted her to find happiness, but not in a psych ward.

CHAPTER FOURTEEN

March 13, 2008

I slept late the morning after we left her at Alhambra, so the first thing I did when I woke up was check my cell phone, expecting there to be a message from a doctor there. But there wasn't. All through that second day, I waited, but a call never came.

We know Janni is all right, because we visit every day. Janni always seems happy. She loves the other girls and they love her. It's like she suddenly has a dozen older sisters. Janni likes the staff, too, because they call her "Miss Tuesday" or whatever day it is.

Susan keeps telling her, "This is just like living in a dorm, Janni. Like when I went away to college."

But it's not. I know Susan is saying that as much for herself, to ease her own pain, as for my benefit, but you go away to college at seventeen or eighteen, not five. If this really were a college dorm, then I could learn to accept it, but she is here because Alhambra is supposed to be helping her. Except nothing is happening. They aren't treating

Janni. She's still on the same medications she was on going in. They're just holding her, and with each passing day it feels like this is becoming our future. I want a doctor. I want several doctors. I want them studying Janni, consulting with each other, and coming up with a plan. I want to know that this incarceration will end.

But the only person who ever meets with us is a social worker. And there is only one doctor here for the entire hospital, Dr. Allen Wingfield. It takes me four days of leaving him messages before he finally calls me back.

"This is Dr. Wingfield. I heard you wanted to speak to me."

"We brought our daughter in about a week ago, so what's the plan?"

"We're still observing her behavior," he replies curtly.

Janni's hospitalization is not turning out how I thought it would. I keep thinking somebody has to recognize what is going on with her. I'm used to doctors having at least some answers. I've always trusted them, because I've never had a reason not to. I got sick, went to the doctor, got a prescription, and got better. Now I am in a world where nobody seems to know anything. This guy is a psychiatrist. He has an MD and years of experience. How can he not have an answer?

"Do you think it is bipolar? That's what Dr. Howe believes now. Have you spoken with her?"

"I have not," he answers simply.

"Don't you think it would be good to talk to her?" I suggest as gently as my emotions will allow. "She's been seeing Janni for three months."

"To be honest, we don't find much benefit talking to the out-patient caregiver," Wingfield replies. "We go by what we see here."

"But that's the problem. You're not seeing it. The hospital is not the real world. She doesn't have to deal with Bodhi."

"I am sure that is true, which is what makes me doubt that she is bipolar or schizophrenic. If she was, I would expect to see a continuation of her symptoms here." Wingfield's tone changes. "By the way, that reminds me. She's been telling the staff and the USC intern who sees her every day that she has schizophrenia. That's not a word your average five-year-old would know," he continues. "Where did she learn that word?"

"She's very smart," I answer. "She has a 146 IQ."

"I get that, but someone had to teach her that word. I asked her what schizophrenia is and she told me it was when you see and hear things other people don't."

"Which is true," I answer.

"Yes, but it is very spot-on for a young child. Have you or your wife told her she has schizophrenia?" he asks pointedly.

"We've been dealing with this for months. One moment she is sweet and the next she is violent and then back to sweet again like nothing happened. So we've been trying to figure out what is going on."

"That doesn't explain how she knows about schizophrenia."

I know where he is going with this. Without a clear answer from doctors, I spend much of my nights on WebMD.com. A year ago I was resistant to Asperger's or autism, but now I look over the symptoms again, trying to find Janni in there. But she isn't. The symptoms don't match. I keep coming back to the page on schizophrenia: *almost complete lack of interest in social relationships, restricted range of emotions or no emotion at all (flat affect).* I think back to Janni saying she "hates" Violet with no passion. *Bizarre behavior, making the person seem 'odd' or 'eccentric' because of unusual mannerisms.* I think of Janni becoming enraged when others dismiss her rats as imaginary. But it is the violence I desperately need to explain. *In active stages of schizophrenia, a person may react with uncontrolled anger or violence to a perceived threat, regardless of how illogical that threat might seem.*

So yes, she's heard us talking about it. What the hell are we supposed to do? This consumes our lives. But if I tell Wingfield this, he will think we are "leading" Janni. We've never "led" Janni anywhere in her life. We've just been trying to keep up.

"It's in our families," I answer instead, which is true.

Wingfield is silent for a moment. Then, "Well, we'll keep observing her."

This is not what I want. I want a plan.

"We just need to control the violence. That's all we need. She's been in for a week and there haven't been any medication changes."

"Because we aren't sure what she might need. She clearly has some issues with controlling her anger. I don't deny that."

"What about Lexapro?"

"What about it?"

"I . . ." I hesitate, wondering how to proceed. "I used to have problems controlling my anger. I would blow up over little insignificant stuff, similar to how she screams and hits when her brother starts crying. I could feel it coming, but I could never stop it."

"Did she ever see any of this?" Wingfield asks.

"Sometimes. Very rarely, but I finally went to a psychiatrist who put me on Lexapro. It does take the edge off for me. I've talked to Dr. Howe about trying it, but she refuses because of the increased risk of suicide."

Wingfield is silent for a moment. "She's right. Antidepressants can increase the risk of suicidal ideation," he finally says.

I've been diagnosed as having chronic depression, but the manifestation of my depression was anger. Maybe it is the same for Janni. Maybe my miracle drug is her miracle drug, too. I'm not really worried about suicide. She's only five, after all.

"But," he continues, "if it works for you, then maybe it will work for her. Let's try it and see if it helps her anger issues."

I feel an immense sense of relief. This may just be the answer. If Janni is just like me and if Lexapro saved me, then it can save her as well.

· · ·

THE NEXT DAY, the sixth day since Janni went in, we arrive but I don't see Janni waiting for us in the hallway like she usually is, waiting for the food we bring since she hardly eats anything from Alhambra's cafeteria.

"Janni?" I call out.

One of the female "technicians," as I have learned they are called, a woman covered in tattoos, approaches us. She looks like she just got out of prison, but she is nice. "She's sleeping in the quiet room." She points to our left.

I know what the "quiet room" is. It's not a patient room. In the old days, they used to call it the "rubber room."

I turn and see Janni through the open door of the room, lying on the bare mattress, her back to us.

"She's sleeping?" Susan asks, surprised. Janni doesn't take naps.

"She was waiting for you all day," the technician tells us, "then about an hour ago she said she wanted to sleep."

"Janni?" I call softly as I enter. The room is spartan, bare of everything except the bed and the sheetless mattress.

She is sleeping deeply. I hate to wake her, but I only have an hour and I am not going to leave without her knowing we were here. I don't want her to think we didn't come.

"Janni, we got Pizza Kitchen for you."

She doesn't stir.

"Janni?" I sit down next to her and touch her back.

No response.

"Janni?" I stand up and come around the other side and see the puddle of drool at the bottom of her sagging mouth, soaking the right side of her face, plastering her hair.

"Janni?" I shake her more urgently.

Nothing. I lift her head, which lolls back and forth in my arms, a deadweight. Her eyes don't move.

"Janni?!" I practically shout. Something is seriously wrong. She is unresponsive. "You stay with her," I say to Susan. "I'm gonna get the nurse."

I run out of the room to the nurses' station. I wait at the counter. I see several staff milling about, but no one seems to notice me.

"Hello?" I call out. It takes everything I have not to hop the counter and wrap my hands around the first throat I reach. I can't do that. I have already learned that these people couldn't care less that this is my daughter. All they care about is their damn rules.

"Hey," I yell now. "We need some help here."

The head nurse comes over.

"Yes?"

"Janni won't wake up."

"She was very tired," she answers in a blasé tone.

"She won't wake up!" I repeat, attempting to drive through this woman's thick skull the fact that this is a medical emergency. "She's lying in a puddle of her own drool! I want a nurse to check her vitals!"

"She's fine. Somebody checks on her every few minutes."

"She was alone when we came in! How do you know she is fine? She's not hooked up to an EKG!"

"She's just tired. It happens."

I'm powerless. Janni may be dying and nobody cares.

"I'm taking her home tonight," I snarl at the nurse. I've had enough of this.

"Well, that's your choice," the nurse says like she doesn't care either way. "But we would need to get permission from the doctor first, and he's already left for the day."

I back away, my fists clenched, desperately wanting to put a hole through the drywall but knowing that would only get me kicked out. Janni is my child, but I have no control over her fate. I'm not a father anymore. I'm a "visitor."

I go back into the quiet room. Susan is gone, probably talking to one of the other girls. I sit down and cradle Janni's head in my lap. I talk to her, repeating "Daddy's here," and telling her I brought her favorite, mac 'n' cheese from California Pizza Kitchen, hoping she will wake up. I touch her chest. I can still feel her heart beating.

Where the hell is Susan? I set Janni's head down and come out of the room, looking for her. I find her sitting in the dining area, talking to a girl. This is the youngest girl I have seen here after Janni. She looks about ten or eleven, but her appearance shocks me. She is wearing a fishnet shirt over a black half top. She looks like a hooker.

Susan turns to me. "This is Carly, Janni's new roommate. Carly, this is my husband, Michael. Tell him what you just told me."

I don't want to listen to some kid. I want a doctor.

"I told you to stay with Janni," I say, barely able to contain my anger. It's not Susan I am angry at, but she is the only one I can get angry with right now.

"I know, but you need to hear this. Carly, tell him."

Carly starts speaking. "Janni was jumping on her bed. I told her to stop because I was afraid she would fall and hurt herself, but she wouldn't listen so I got the staff. She wouldn't listen to them, either. She started climbing the curtains, saying she could fly."

"She was literally climbing the walls," Susan says, giving me a pointed look.

"Then she was climbing on the furniture and jumping off," Carly continues.

Susan shakes her head at me. "It's the Lexapro. I know it. It's winding her up just like the Ritalin did."

I feel an incredible sense of despair. I was convinced the Lexapro would work. I arrogantly assumed that because it worked for me it would work her. Instead, it's left her like this.

"The staff couldn't get her to stop, so they gave her an injection."

An injection?

"What injection?" I demand.

"I don't know, but it still didn't work, so they gave her a second one."

Susan gives me the same pointed look. "When I called in earlier and asked how she was doing, they told me she was fine."

"No, it was pretty scary," Carly interjects. "She's a cool girl, though. I really like her."

The head nurse suddenly appears. "Carly, go to the community room," she commands sternly. Carly immediately runs off. The nurse leans in close to us and lowers her voice. "I have to ask you to refrain from talking to other patients."

"They're the only ones telling us what's going on with our daughter," Susan shoots back.

"If you have a question, you can come to me."

"Janni got an injection?" I ask.

The nurse's hostility and dislike of us is barely contained.

"I will check the logbook." The "logbook" is a gigantic three-ring binder that contains the treatment information for each patient. "In the meantime, if you continue to disregard our rules regarding respecting patient privacy, you will have to leave."

I can't believe this. "You mean we couldn't see our daughter?"

"Not if you can't respect our rules."

There is no doubt. We are being threatened. And I can tell from her demeanor that it is not an empty threat. Whatever they think is wrong with Janni, they clearly don't see us as part of the solution.

"Now, if you will give me a minute, I will check the logbook." The nurse walks off to the nurses' station.

We follow and wait.

After what feels like an eternity, the nurse returns with the log-book, so big she can barely carry it. She sets it down on the counter and begins flipping through it until she finds Janni's file.

"It says she was not following directions so she received an IM of Benadryl."

"For what?" I ask.

"It says here she was not following directions."

"What was she doing?" I ask.

"She was climbing the walls!" Susan shouts before the nurse can answer.

The nurse placidly reads the report. "I don't see anything here about climbing the walls."

"Because nobody logs anything around here," Susan fires back. "I called several times today and every time I was told Janni was doing fine."

"What time did this happen?" I ask, trying to remain calm so we don't get tossed. I am more afraid of getting barred from seeing Janni now than anything else.

The nurse reads some more. "It says she received the first IM around noon and then another at two."

"What does 'IM' mean?" I ask.

"Intramuscular. An injection into the muscles."

Rage erupts into my veins. In my mind, I visualize them holding the screaming and struggling Janni down and injecting her.

"Where?"

"Where, what?" The nurse is confused.

"Where was she injected?" I say, my voice slow, deliberate, a by-product of trying to control my rage. They are sticking my little girl with needles.

"We usually give it in the bottom."

I grab on to the edge of the table to keep my hands from lashing out at this nurse. They held her down *and* pulled down her pants and shot her in the butt?

"Why?" I manage to ask. "Why not just give her a pill?"

"Usually it is because the patient won't take oral medication."

This doesn't sound like Janni. She's been popping pills for three months now.

"How long will she be like this? Is she okay?"

"She is fine. We check on her."

"We want her off the Lexapro," Susan says. "That is what is causing this."

"You will have to take that up with the doctor," the nurse replies.

"Wingfield takes days to return our calls," I respond.

"He is very busy," the nurse replies coldly.

"We want her off the Lexapro right now," Susan demands.

An idea pops into my head. "Before she could get the Lexapro, I had to sign a piece of paper giving permission. If I gave permission, I can revoke it."

The nurse looks at me, clearly annoyed. *Yeah,* I think, *you aren't used to parents who know their rights.*

"So you want to pull authorization for the Lexapro?" she finally says.

"Yes. Effective immediately. Give me the sheet and I will sign it right now."

"Just a minute." The nurse retreats back into the nurses' station. I'm still angry, but for the first time today I feel some measure of being in control again. I left Janni here, expecting that my energy would be directed at fighting whatever is going on with her. Instead, I am spending more time fighting with the Alhambra staff.

The nurse returns with the medication authorization sheet and I check the box next to "*I DO NOT give permission for this medication to be administered to my child.*"

"Just so you know," the nurse says to us while I sign my name, "this would be considered refusing treatment. If you do this, the doctor may release her on the grounds that you refused to comply with his recommendations."

I stare at her, hating her guts. Once again, we are being threatened.

I go back into the quiet room. Janni is still passed out. I sit down next to her and cradle her head in my arms, telling her "Daddy is here." They say that the subconscious remembers everything. I hope this is true and she hears me.

CHAPTER FIFTEEN

March 21, 2008

Janni is being discharged today. She has been here at Alhambra for almost two weeks and we have come to visit her every day, driving forty miles each way, spending a total of four hours in traffic to see Janni for one hour, assuming she is actually conscious when we get there and not knocked out by injections of Benadryl, which have become an almost daily occurrence.

Every day I walk in with the same hope: that I will see a noticeable change in Janni. But that is not really what I am looking for. Her violence in here has never approached her violence at home. It decreased the moment she came in, either because she no longer had to deal with Bodhi or because she had finally found kids she felt comfortable with, even if those "kids" were mostly teenagers.

Over the past two weeks, Susan has spoken to every girl in this place, questioning them about their younger days, trying to find out if any were like Janni, and in particular if they had Janni's "imagination." We keep referring to it as her "imagination" even though it has become obvious that her imaginary friends rule her world and she talks about them like they are real. They seem to have a life of their own. But none of the girls, not even that boy Susan met on the first day who said, "She has what I have," are or have ever been like Janni in that way. None of them live most of their lives in a complete fantasy world.

So one of the things I look for every time I come is for Janni to be more aware of what is happening to her. I look at Janni's eyes now every time I see her. I never paid much attention to eyes. Hell, I dated Susan for years without being able to remember the color of her eyes (hazel). But since the violence began, I've had a lot of experience holding Janni down to keep her from hitting or kicking Bodhi, so I've had the opportunity to look Janni in the eyes a lot. When I do, I don't see them looking back at me. They look blind, like the entire world has disappeared. I have a photo of Janni that I use as the desktop image on our computer. It was taken sometime in the spring before she turned two. She is at a park with the setting sun behind her, illuminating her blond hair into wisps of gold. She is looking at the camera and smiling. Not an exaggerated smile like kids do when you tell them you are going to take their picture, but an acknowledging half smile. Susan took the picture before Janni had time to react, so this photograph is an image of Janni, frozen in time. Every time I boot up the computer, Janni's eyes appear, looking right at me. There is warmth in them along with a simple look of happiness.

For three years I have been hoping to see those eyes again.

There is another photo. One Sara took as we left Violet's birthday party. In it, Janni's face is expressionless, devoid of emotion. Looking back at that photo now, I can see what I missed then: There is no emotion in her eyes. When I come to visit Janni, I don't expect a return to those eyes of three years ago at the park. All I am looking for is a softening of her expression into an actual emotion. I'm looking for some sense of the rebirth of peace. This is what I wanted Alhambra to fix. But they didn't.

Janni is leaving on the same medications she came in on: Seroquel, an antipsychotic, and Depakote, a mood stabilizer.

I look down at the discharge summary. Next to "Diagnosis" is simply "Mood Disorder NOS," meaning "not otherwise specified." Meaning Wingfield doesn't know what is wrong with our daughter. After two weeks, we are right back where we started.

Three days ago, I got a letter in the mail from Blue Cross, Susan's health insurance, addressed to "January Schofield." When I opened it, the letter read, "After careful review, authorization for further inpatient days is denied, based on one or more of the following criteria:"

1. *The patient no longer meets the criteria for acute psychiatric hospitalization as per your* Blue Cross Patient Handbook.

The requirements for acute psychiatric inpatient care are that the patient must be an *immediate* (meaning in this exact moment in time) threat to him/herself or others. The fact that Janni has continued to react violently to Bodhi's crying, forcing us to leave visiting hours early, apparently does not qualify, since Janni has not articulated an actual plan to harm him.

2. *The patient is not responding to the current course of treatment.*

Apparently, if you have a psychiatric illness, you better hope the first course of treatment is the right one. Somehow, I don't think Blue

Cross would say this to a child with leukemia who hadn't responded to the first round of chemotherapy.

3. *The patient is not improving and there is no reasonable expectation of the patient making a recovery or improving beyond his/her current status.*

I pick up the phone and call Blue Cross, asking, "So what are we supposed to do?"

"You can take her to a state hospital," the soulless woman on the other end replies.

"There are no state hospitals anymore," I inform her. Former California governor Pete Wilson closed the last state psychiatric hospital, Camarillo State Hospital, in 1998. Ironically, the former Camarillo State Hospital is now the newest campus of the California State University system, the very same university system I work for. There are a handful of places with "State Hospital" after their name, but these are actually prisons for sex offenders, not psychiatric facilities.

The woman on the other end of the line has no answer for me.

Janni is being released not because she's gotten over whatever it is that brought her to this place, but because the insurance company won't pay anymore.

I turn to Janni, who is waiting in the hallway with her Disney Princess roller suitcase.

"You ready to come home?" I ask, looking for anything in her demeanor that shows change.

"Yep," she answers. I see no gravity in her face, no appreciation of her impending freedom.

"You got Hero? We wouldn't want to leave him here."

"I got him. Where are we going to eat?"

"Well, since this is a special day, I thought we'd go to Pizza Kitchen."

"How long will it take to get there?"

"Well, there's gonna be some traffic right now. It might take us an hour or so."

Janni screams.

I look to Susan, who quickly covers Bodhi's three-month-old ears with her hands. She looks up at me, naked fear on her face. We lived without this for two weeks and didn't realize how much of a vacation it was.

The nurse cuts in. "Janni. What did I tell you? No screaming."

"Fine," Janni says, sulkily. "But I don't want to deal with Bodhi's crying."

I look at the discharge nurse. "Are you sure she's ready to be released?"

"You have to allow for readjustment time," the nurse replies, reading our faces.

It's almost evening and the sun is setting as we walk back to the car. I close my eyes, enjoying the warmth of the sun on my face.

I open my eyes and look at Janni. Her face is blank, her head down, plodding along pulling her suitcase.

We reach our car and I load her bag. When I put my hands on the rear hatch to close it, I realize they are shaking. I'm terrified of my own daughter, of the first explosion of violence I can still sense in Janni, waiting to erupt.

I pull my hands down and rub them roughly together. I have to get control of my emotions. I have become "shell-shocked," living for so long in constant fear of Janni hurting Bodhi that I can't remember ever not feeling this way.

Janni opens the front passenger door and climbs in.

"Janni, you need to sit in the back," I say. "It's the law."

"No," Janni answers.

"Janni, get in the backseat," I repeat, trying to sound commanding but hearing the fear in my voice.

"I don't want to," Janni answers.

"Let it go," Susan tells me.

"No," I reply, trying to sound stronger than I feel. "She needs to do what we say."

"It's fine," Susan answers, already in the backseat. "I'm tired. I want to go home."

I look at Susan, wanting her to back me up, but also understanding. I don't really care if Janni wants to sit in the front. Like Susan, all I really want is peace. I just want us to go home.

As I load Bodhi's car seat into the car, a distinct odor reaches me. I'm going to have to change Bodhi. He cries in the car anyway, but a dirty diaper will only make it worse. When Janni was an infant, she never seemed to care.

I take Bodhi out of his car seat and gently lay him down in the grass in front of the car to change him.

"I want to go," Janni calls from inside the car.

"Janni, can you bring me the wipes?"

"I'm hungry!" she yells.

"Janni, I have to change him. I never left you in a poopie. I always changed you right away." I want her to understand that everything I do for Bodhi I also did for her.

Janni reluctantly gets out of the car and brings me the wipes. She remains standing by me as I change Bodhi. I feel a rush of hope. This is what I want, her beside me.

"I'll go throw it away," Susan calls, getting out of the car.

"No, I will." I hand her the freshly diapered Bodhi and stand up. There is a dumpster in the far corner of the parking lot.

I start walking and light a cigarette. I have to be calm for the drive home. It's going to be a long one.

I come back to the car and climb in the driver's side.

Bodhi begins to cry.

Instantly, every nerve in my body goes on full alert. I watch Janni. For a second she doesn't react. Then she puts her hands over her ears and screams, "Bodhi! Stop crying!"

"Janni!" I call, warning her, my voice threatening. "You want to go to Pizza Kitchen, right?"

"He won't stop crying!"

"Janni, we're not going anywhere until I know you're going to be okay with Bodhi."

"Make him stop crying!" she says to Susan, almost begging, as if she really believes Susan can stop it.

"If you want him to stop crying, why don't you play with him?" I say. "Entertain him."

She grabs a bottle of water next to her.

I put my hand over the bottle of water. "Janni, if you throw that at him, we are not going to Pizza Kitchen!" I say, staring at her, hoping she'll accept my threat and back down.

She lets go of the water bottle. I relax. "Good girl," I say, turning back to the steering column and putting on my seat belt.

Out of the corner of my eye, I see Janni take off her shoe. I grab for it, but the seat belt won't let me reach. Janni turns around in her seat, gets up on her knees, and throws the shoe back. Susan knocks it away.

I release my seat belt and grab Janni's other shoe. Janni starts looking around for something to throw.

"Janni, sit down!" I command. The fear is gone, replaced by adrenaline. I am back in battle.

Janni ignores me and reaches for her CD cases to throw. I take them from her. As I do, she hits me and screams again.

"She wasn't ready to be released," Susan cries from the back.

"I know that!" I snap. "What do you expect me to do about it?"

"She needs to go back!"

"No! We are not going back! She is part of this family and she has to learn to follow our rules!" I reach past Janni and open her door. "Get out," I order.

Janni looks at me, that same evil grin on her face. "No."

"Get out!" I say again. "When you calm down, you can get back in this car."

She doesn't move. Instead, she's staring at me, grinning, daring me to pull her out.

So I do. I get out and go around and pull her out onto the pavement, where she sits down like a sullen child.

I go to the back of the car and get Hero Bear out of her suitcase. "Here, hold Hero." I hold her bear out to her. "When Bodhi cries, just squeeze Hero Bear." I realize I'm ping-ponging back and forth between treating her like the child she is and treating her like the angry teenager she might actually be. I don't know who she is.

Janni takes Hero from me. But instead of hugging him to her, she starts yanking at his head.

"Janni, what are you doing?"

"Trying to pull his head off."

"Don't do that!"

I take Hero from her. She grabs him back and pitches him into the parking lot.

"Janni, why did you do that?"

"I don't want him anymore. He's a bad bear."

"She's not ready to go," Susan says again.

Suddenly, Janni reaches in through the still-open front passenger door and starts throwing anything she can get her hands on into the parking lot. The contents of the front of the car are piling up on the asphalt behind me.

Bodhi is still crying. Janni moves to the rear passenger door, Bodhi's door, and starts to open it. Inside, I see Susan immediately put herself over Bodhi. I grab Janni and pull her back, away from the car.

"She needs to go back!" Susan screams at me. "How long are you going to wait? Until she kills him? Do you think those idiots back in there," she points to Alhambra, "will care if she kills Bodhi? They'll just say 'Oh, well.'"

I know. I should have brought both cars, I think angrily to myself, but I decided on one car, to have us ride as a family, to prove to myself that we could function normally. But Janni has been out for thirty minutes and we can't even make it out of the parking lot. This is not going to work.

"Come on, Janni," I say, defeated. "Let's go."

Janni immediately stops trying to hit Susan and Bodhi and looks up at me. "Where are we going?"

"Back inside."

Janni doesn't protest. I pick Hero up off the pavement and hand him to her. This time she hugs him to her. I get her suitcase out of the back of the car.

Susan follows, Bodhi in her arms, as we retrace the steps we walked forty minutes ago. It is a walk of shame.

I pick up the phone outside the gate.

"Nursing," comes the answer on the other end.

"It's Michael Schofield. We're still here. We never made it out of the parking lot. Janni has been hitting and screaming the whole time."

"So what do you want us to do?" the woman replies, sounding confused, like this has never happened before.

"We're bringing her back."

"But she's already been discharged!"

"I realize that, but nothing has changed. She is still violent."

"Just a minute."

I wait. The discharge nurse who walked us out comes on the line. "What's going on?"

"Nothing's changed, that's what's going on. She's still as violent as ever."

"I told you it would take time for her to get readjusted."

"We can't even get home," I reply.

The nurse sighs. "We'll be right out."

We wait. Janni is calm now. The nurse comes out with one of the technicians.

"What's going on, Janni?"

Janni suddenly kicks at Susan, while trying to reach up and hit Bodhi. Susan lifts him clear.

"Whoa, Janni!" the tech says, moving forward to take her by the shoulders. "You can't do that."

"I am going to get scissors and cut off my feet!" Janni announces.

All of us fall silent, stunned.

"Why do you want to do that?" the nurse asks.

"Because then I can't kick Mommy and Bodhi." She is breathing heavily from the exertion of fighting to get free from the tech, her eyes still fixed on Susan and Bodhi.

Everything goes dead inside me . . . all the anger and frustration. I feel nothing. Behind me, I can hear Susan break into a sob.

"Okay, Janni," the nurse says. "Come with me." She holds out her hand.

Janni abruptly stops fighting against the technician and calmly takes the nurse's hand with Hero in her other as they turn toward the adolescent unit, looking like a child happily going off with her mother.

Except that her mother is sobbing behind me.

"Janni," I call, still not sure if I'm doing the right thing.

She twists back, still walking away. "It's okay, Mommy and Daddy. Just bring me my food and visit me at visiting hours."

WE DRIVE HOME in the darkness, the seat beside me empty. Susan is in the back with Bodhi, who has thankfully fallen asleep as we ride in silence. I can hear her sobbing softly. I know I need to comfort her, but I don't know what to say. There is no comfort.

Finally, Susan calls her mother.

"She said she wanted to cut her feet off," Susan cries into the phone. "She wanted to go back. She knew she wasn't ready to come home, so she told them what she knew would get her back in." Susan chokes on a sob. "She's happy there."

I drive, listening to the only side of the conversation I can hear.

"I feel like I'm losing my daughter," Susan cries to her mother. "And there's nothing I can do."

This is exactly how I feel, powerless. I thought I could fix Janni, but whatever is going on inside her mind is stronger than me.

I want to take Susan in my arms, but not because I want to comfort her. There is no comforting. This is hell. I want to grab on to Susan to stop myself from slipping under. My heart is ripping apart. We're losing our daughter.

I need to cry, too, more than I've ever needed to cry in my life. I can feel the tears forming, burning the edges of my eyes, blurring my vision. I open my mouth to let the sob out, but all that comes out is something that sounds like I am choking.

It won't come.

I've never been afraid to show emotion. But for some reason it won't come. My vision starts to clear. The tears are disappearing. The rock in my chest begins to fade.

I am changing. I regrip the steering wheel, refocused on my driving. The pain is gone, replaced by nothing but the determination to keep this family going, no matter what it takes. Maybe because Susan is a sobbing wreck in the backseat and Janni still needs someone to fight for her and figure out what is going on. Or maybe it's because I still have to go to work tomorrow, stand in front of a classroom, and teach like none of this is happening.

CHAPTER SIXTEEN

March 24, 2008

Wingfield was on vacation when Janni was released from Alhambra. When he returns and finds her back, he calls me.

"Frankly," he tells me over the phone (we've still never met face-to-face), "I was surprised to see her back. She was doing so well."

I don't bother pointing out that there was no way he could know that since he was on vacation a full week before Janni was released, so I simply tell him what happened.

After listening, he says, "I'd like to try Ritalin again."

It takes a few seconds to comprehend this. My dad has always told me that the definition of insanity is doing the same thing over and over again but expecting different results.

"We told you what happened when she was on Ritalin," I answer, trying to keep my voice even. "It wound her up just like the Lexapro and she got even more violent." I can't for the life of me understand why he wants to try it again. I know from talking to Dr. Howe that she hasn't been able to share Janni's medical history because he won't return her calls.

"I know that's what you said," he replies, "but you also said you only gave her two doses before you stopped it. I would like to try it again and go a little longer this time, give it more of a chance."

I have been progressively losing faith in doctors, though I've still never outright said no to any of them. But I don't trust Wingfield.

"No. We've already tried Ritalin and it didn't work. It sped up her heart rate and made her bounce off the walls. I'm not giving authorization for Ritalin. What about other drugs, other antipsychotics?"

"I'm not sure she needs another antipsychotic. What I'm seeing are not symptoms of psychosis."

"Look, I won't sign authorization for Ritalin," I tell him. I don't see what he can do. He can't use the threat that Blue Cross will deny authorization for further inpatient stays, because I've already gotten a letter from them saying that. We're now paying for Alhambra out of pocket. The only reason she's still at Alhambra is for me to buy enough time until I can get her into UCLA, which is where we want her. Alhambra clearly doesn't have a clue. UCLA is a teaching hospital, but it's not "in-network" for Susan's Blue Cross plan.

When I first became a lecturer at CSUN, I was offered health insurance but turned it down because we had Susan's, but when I explained the situation to my benefits coordinator at work, I discovered that if we terminated Susan's insurance, leaving us with no insurance at all, I could enroll in one of the plans offered by CSUN immediately without having to wait for open enrollment. I took the booklet containing health plans and called each of them, searching for one that had UCLA in-network. A Blue Shield HMO did. Susan sent off the letter to Blue Cross, terminating our coverage on March 31. The next day, April 1, my insurance will kick in and we can get Janni into UCLA. April 1 is only eight days away. I hate that I have to leave Janni in this hellhole for another eight days, but I don't see any other way. I can't bring her home when she is still a risk to Bodhi.

"That's true," Wingfield says, "I do need your approval, but if you won't allow me to treat Janni, then I can't justify keeping her. I would have no choice but to release her."

"But she's not better," I protest. "If you release her, what are we supposed to do? She is still a major threat to the safety of her little brother!"

"It wouldn't be my choice," he replies coldly. "There are a lot of kids waiting for beds, and if you're not going to allow me to treat her as I see fit, then I would have no choice but to discharge her immediately."

"When?"

"Today."

There have been plenty of doctors in my life that I didn't like. But what I feel for Wingfield is more than simple dislike. He has become the enemy. I have two choices: either let him give Janni a drug I know will make her worse, or let her come home and possibly hurt or kill Bodhi.

I look over at Bodhi, sleeping peacefully.

"I give my permission," I finally say, my voice quiet.

"Great," he says. "I'll go ahead and give the order to start today. When you come in for visiting hours tonight, there will be an authorization sheet waiting for you."

BEFORE WE ARE let onto the girls' unit, we are told to check in at the nurses' station. The head nurse, a woman whose unpleasant personality reminds me of Nurse Ratched from *One Flew Over the Cuckoo's Nest*, comes over with a piece of paper.

"The doctor left this for you to sign," she says. "It is an authorization for Ritalin . . ."

"I know what it is," I reply bluntly and quickly sign it.

111

The nurse nods to the technician, who lets us in. "Janni's asleep," the technician tells us. "In there." She points to the quiet room.

Janni is lying down on the bare mattress. But is she asleep or knocked out? I go into the room. "Janni? Daddy's here."

Janni doesn't move. I kneel down by her. Her hair is mangled and plastered over her face. I brush it back and see a familiar stream of drool. I lean in very close to feel her breathe, to know she is still alive.

I get up and charge out to the nurses' station. I don't panic anymore. I just want to know what the hell happened, because they never call us. Out of the corner of my eye, I see Susan slipping off toward Janni's roommate to ask her. Thankfully, Nurse Ratched takes so long to come over that she doesn't see Susan do this.

"Yes?" she asks, annoyed, as if I am pointlessly interrupting her.

"Janni's knocked out again," I say, making little effort to hide my hostility.

To my surprise, Nurse Ratched doesn't claim she has to check the logbook.

"She refused to go to group therapy and started hitting the staff," the nurse says.

I sigh, my fists clenched. "Of course she did. It's because of the Ritalin. I told Wingfield it would make her worse, but he wouldn't listen."

The nurse is completely unsympathetic.

"Well, that is something you will have to take up with the doctor. We had to give her two PRNs of Thorazine."

Thorazine. My blood turns cold. I've read about Thorazine. It is an old antipsychotic, no longer used very much. In the old days it was used to sedate violent patients.

"Why not Benadryl?" I demand.

"Benadryl is used when a patient is noncooperative. When they are violent and pose a risk to staff and other patients, we use Thorazine."

This can't be reality. This can't be really happening.

I turn away. I have to. If I don't, I will do something bad.

I go into the room. Susan is back, lying next to Janni.

"It's the Ritalin," she says. "They gave her the Ritalin and she went nuts again."

"I know," I reply and sit down next to Janni. I smell urine. I move her top leg over and see a stain on her pants between her legs. She peed herself and they left her in it. She is also wearing the same clothes she was wearing yesterday.

"Janni?" I call. She stirs, her arm flopping over. I say her name several more times, telling her I am here, before she sits up. She looks around the room, her eyes vacant and seemingly unable to focus.

"Janni?"

She turns to me, her eyes droopy. Her hair is wild and frizzy. She flops down again.

I lift her back up. "Janni, why are you wearing the same clothes from yesterday?"

She looks down at herself. "I didn't have any clean clothes," she answers, like she doesn't really care.

"Janni, are you taking baths here?" Susan asks.

"No," she answers, trying to go back to sleep, but I hold her up. "They don't have baths here, only showers."

"So are you taking a shower?" Susan asks.

"Sometimes," Janni answers, groggily.

Susan brushes Janni's hair with her hand. "Is somebody helping you wash your hair?"

"No," Janni slurs.

"Why not?" Susan asks.

"Nobody will come in with me. They say I have to do it by myself."

"So your hair hasn't been washed?"

Janni shakes her head.

"She needs a shower," Susan says to me. "I'll go to her room and get her clean clothes, shampoo, and a brush."

"We're not supposed to go in their rooms," I remind her.

"I don't care," Susan answers firmly. "They're not taking care of her, so screw it."

I can't argue with that.

"I don't want a shower," Janni says, weakly.

Normally, I would let it go. Janni has never been that concerned over her hygiene, but I want her to care. I know she's only five, but not caring about hygiene is the first step on the road to becoming one of the adults I see here every day, wearing pajamas in the middle of the day.

"Janni, you need a shower. We'll make it quick. Come on." I stand up.

"I can't walk," Janni whines.

"Then I'll carry you. But you are getting a shower and clean clothes."

There is a bathroom right here in the quiet room. I pull the handle, but it is locked.

I leave Janni on the bed and go up to the tattooed tech. "I need to give Janni a shower."

"Showers are in the morning," she tells me.

"She peed herself. I need to give her a shower and a change of clothes."

The technician turns to see Susan coming out of Janni's room with shampoo, a brush, and a change of clothes.

"You can't be back there," the tech calls.

"You're not taking care of her," Susan replies, "so we have to."

The tech looks from Susan to me. I sense her realization that we're not backing down.

"Okay." She sighs. "There's a shower in the bathroom of the quiet room. I can unlock it for you."

Susan musters some politeness. "Thank you."

"You know we're not supposed to do this," the tech tells us as she unlocks the doors.

"I'm going to need towels, too," I tell her. I couldn't care less whether this tech gets into trouble. I will not leave my daughter like this.

"Okay." She heads away to get them.

"Janni," Susan asks, "do you want Mommy or Daddy to give you a shower?"

"Daddy," Janni answers.

The tech comes back with the towels. "Thanks," I say.

"Come on, Janni." I usher Janni into the bathroom.

As I start to close the door behind me, the tech calls, "Wait. You're going in there with her?" I look back at her and she looks alarmed.

"She won't bathe herself. I have to do it for her or it won't get done," I say, closing the door.

I turn on the shower and hold my hand under the water until I feel the temperature is right. "Okay, Janni, get undressed."

"I can't," she whines.

"Fine." I get down on my knees. "Put your hand on my shoulder," I tell her. I am afraid if she doesn't hold on to me she'll fall over lifting her leg to get her pants off.

I get her clothes off and she climbs under the water. I wash her hair. It is incredibly matted, and I take a brush to work through the thick globs of hair.

"Ow!" She pulls her head away. She hates getting her hair brushed.

"Janni, I have to get the tangles."

"But it hurts!"

I am about to argue with her. Then I think, forget it. She has been through enough today. I rub some soap into the washcloth and go over her body. She just stands there.

"Turn around so the soap gets washed off," I tell her. I have to tell her to do everything. Susan and I take turns taking care of Janni's hygiene at home, but this feels different. We are in a psychiatric hospital. I feel a sudden sense of fear, wondering if I will be doing this when Janni is an adult.

I turn off the shower and dry her down. I help her into her underwear and nightgown.

I open the door to the bathroom. Janni walks out and I come out behind her, happy to get back out into the cool air.

"What do you want to do now, Janni?" I ask. "Do you want to eat?"

"I want to go back to bed."

"I'll take her back to her room and tuck her in bed. I've got Hero," Susan says.

"Okay." I give Janni a kiss. "Love you, sweetie."

She doesn't respond.

I watch them go and wheel Bodhi's stroller into the hallway to wait for Susan.

Nurse Ratched is waiting for me, glaring. "I was told you insisted on giving Janni a shower, even after my staff told you no," she says, staring right at me, her voice cold.

At first, I think that must be what the tech said to save her sorry job.

"She was lying in her own urine," I reply. "Would you leave your child like that until morning?"

Nurse Ratched doesn't blink. "My staff member told me that she told you that was not allowed, but you ignored her, demanding to give Janni a shower."

I am about to say, *Well, how do you think we got the towels if* your staff member *was so against us giving Janni a shower?* but the tone of her voice finally sinks into my brain. Something is wrong, I know, but I'm too tired and angry to figure it out.

"I would ask that you not give Janni any more showers while she's here," she says, then walks away.

WE GET HOME at nine-thirty. I didn't want to make dinner, but Susan is hungry, so I do it while Susan gives Bodhi a bath.

She is in the tub with him, like I do when I give him a bath. We got a baby bathtub for Janni but never used it, so we didn't bother getting one for Bodhi. It is easier just to get in there with them.

I am washing the dishes when I hear a hard knock at the door. Honey leaps up from her slumber and goes crazy, barking at the door.

I turn to look at the clock on the stove. Ten-thirty. There is only one group of people who come knocking on your door at ten-thirty at night.

"There's somebody at the door," I call to Susan in the bathroom as I dry my hands on a hand towel and neatly fold it.

"Who?" she calls back.

I already know, even before I make it to the door to look through the peephole and see a Hispanic man with a clipboard and an ID badge hanging around his neck. On either side of him are two Los Angeles County sheriff's deputies. On some level, I've been expecting this ever since I saw the look of distrust on Nurse Ratched's face earlier tonight.

"You need to get dressed," I call to Susan.

She comes out of the bathroom, holding Bodhi, both dripping wet. "What? Who is it?"

"Just get some clothes on," I reply calmly.

She darts into the bedroom and closes the door. I grab Honey's collar and open the door.

"Hello," the Hispanic man says to me. Honey is barking and trying to lunge at them. The man has to shout to be heard over her barking.

"Sorry to bother you so late. Are you," he looks down at his notes, "Michael Schofield?"

"Yes." Strangely, I feel completely calm, even peaceful. I feel no fear. Maybe it is because I have no control over what will happen now.

"You're the father of January Schofield?" he asks.

"Yes."

"Is your wife," he checks his notes again, "Susan, here?"

"She's in the bedroom getting dressed. She just gave our son a bath."

"She is the biological mother of January?"

"Yes."

He is writing on his clipboard. "Can we come in?"

I find it funny that he actually asked. It's not like I could say no.

"Sure." I back up, pulling Honey with me. "Sorry about our dog. She is very territorial."

Susan comes out in her bathrobe. To my great annoyance, she hasn't tied the sash very tight and the robe falls open, pretty much exposing her. I wanted her to put on some real clothes. She's going to need them. Bodhi is not dressed at all, still naked in her arms.

"Are you Mrs. Schofield?" the man asks, his face betraying no reaction to the fact that Susan is basically flashing him, albeit unintentionally.

"Yes," Susan answers, looking like a deer in headlights.

"My name is Carlos and I'm a field investigator for the Department of Child and Family Services. I will need to talk to both of you."

"Okay," Susan answers, looking from me to Carlos and back again, remaining where she is, like she expects Carlos to start telling us why he's here. *Wow*, I think, *she really is clueless.* She doesn't know what is happening. She doesn't get that Carlos expects Susan to invite him someplace where they can talk in private away from me, because that's what they do. I have seen enough episodes of *Law & Order: Special Victims Unit* to know how this works.

Realizing that Susan didn't understand his tactful request, Carlos tries again. "Mrs. Schofield, is there somewhere we can speak in private?"

He looks at me. "You don't mind, do you?"

I shake my head. "Not at all."

He nods. "I am going to need to talk to you as well, Mr. Schofield, and then both of you together, but I want to start with Mrs. Schofield first."

Of course you do, I think to myself. He wants to isolate Susan to see if he can get her to confess to knowing that something is happening. That's how they work.

"The bedroom," Susan answers, suddenly snapping out of her paralysis. Carlos and my mostly naked wife enter the bedroom. Carlos closes the door behind him.

I turn back to the deputies. I am still holding on to Honey's collar to prevent her from lunging and nipping them. If they are going to arrest me, I need to put Honey away.

"Listen, do you mind if I take Honey down to our garage?" I ask the nearest deputy, a huge, hulking fellow.

He looks at Honey. "Sure." He steps aside to let us pass. "You're not going to run, are you?" he says as I open the door.

I look back at him. He is smiling, like he is joking, but I know he isn't. They think I molested my own daughter. I am sure he would love me to run, so that when he caught me he could legally use that nice baton hanging from his belt on me.

"No, I'm not going to run."

"Okay, then. Make it quick."

I take Honey downstairs to our garage. I keep a spare drinking bowl down here and extra bottles of water. I take one and fill the bowl. I don't know when, or if, I will be back, so I want to make sure Honey has water. I give her what might be a final pat and kiss on her nose and close the door. I can still hear her barking as I come upstairs, reentering the apartment.

The second deputy is walking around our place, picking things up and putting them down. I know he's searching. What does he expect to find? Child pornography?

"You don't mind if we look around?" the bigger deputy asks me, even though they already are.

"Go right ahead." I don't care. I have nothing to hide.

Okay, I think to myself, *what to do now?* I look around the apartment, trying to prioritize. I feel extremely focused. What will make Susan's life easier when they take me?

I return to washing the dishes.

I see the other deputy pause over the coffee table and pick up the lid of a game called Feed the Kitty. Of course, "kitty" is a slang term for the female anatomy. Except that this game has a real kitty and the goal is to prevent the kitty from eating your mice. You roll the dice to see how many mice you have to feed the kitty. The player with the most mice at the end wins.

The deputy, apparently realizing the game has no sexual connotations, puts the lid down.

I hear Susan cry out. That rattles me. I wasn't expecting that. Does she actually believe whatever Carlos is telling her? How could she?

The bedroom door opens and Carlos comes out with Bodhi in his arms.

"Would you mind holding him for a minute?" he asks me.

"Uh, sure," I reply, taking Bodhi from him. I find this strange. If he thinks I am a child molester, why is he handing me Bodhi? Through the open bedroom door I can see Susan sitting on the bed, hunched over, sobbing, her bathrobe completely fallen open, showing off everything.

"Thanks," Carlos says to me. "I was worried your wife might drop him. She's pretty upset."

He goes back into the bedroom, closing the door. *Well, so much for trying to get things cleaned up,* I think.

I go over to our rocking chair and sit down, cradling Bodhi in my arms. I start to gently rock him, just like I did over five years ago when Janni was a baby.

Back then, I never would have imagined any of this happening.

I look down at Bodhi, enjoying the weight and warmth of his body. It feels like I am holding him for the first time all over again. Maybe because this might be the last time I ever get to hold him. I know I didn't sexually molest Janni. But I also know I can't prove that, which is, I suppose, why I'm not angry. These deputies are here to arrest me on suspicion of child molestation. They will take me to the local station to be booked, and then I will be transported to the "Twin Towers," the main LA County Jail, to await my hearing. Not that I will make it to my hearing. I know what happens to child molesters in prison. I've seen TV shows on prison life. Any prisoner would be only too happy to take me out. I will be walking somewhere and suddenly be attacked, shanked, stabbed repeatedly, to ensure no chance of saving me in the infirmary. By my reckoning, I will be dead by the end of the week. Oddly, the idea of being stabbed to death, of death itself, doesn't bother me at all. All I care about is Janni. And that is the only reason I don't want to die. Janni will be devastated. What will her life be like from this point on? The only thing I am afraid of is that if I'm gone, any chance for Janni's future will die with me. She will gradually become lost. If I could trust somebody else to make sure Janni would be okay, I would be fine with dying. I put my cheek against Bodhi's. He's so young that he won't even remember me. But Janni will. How will she be able to forget me? I snuggle with Bodhi. I love him so much. He is a beautiful boy.

Suddenly, I want to cry. His life seems so brutally unfair. He is being screwed out of everything. But once again, the tears seem to get stuck before they can come out.

The bedroom door opens and Susan comes out. Her eyes are red. She wipes them and reaches out for Bodhi.

"What's going on?" I ask as if I don't know.

"He'll tell you" is all she replies. It bothers me that her head is down and she won't look me in the eye.

I hand Bodhi to her and stand up. Carlos is waiting for me at the bedroom door. I walk into the bedroom, the big deputy following me. He shuts the door and stands in front of it, arms crossed.

Carlos looks over his notes for a moment and then looks up at me.

"Okay, Mr. Schofield, I'm really sorry about the hour and interrupting your dinner." He appears to be genuinely contrite, which seems strange since he's supposedly talking to a man who molested his own daughter. "Do you have any idea why we're here?"

I see no need to beat around the bush, to pretend like I don't know. "I'm guessing it's because I've been accused of abuse of some sort."

Carlos gives me a sharp look. "What makes you think that?"

Because I'm not an idiot, I want to say.

"Why else would you be here?" I reply instead.

Carlos appears to consider this, then returns to his clipboard.

"Makes sense. How often do you give her a bath?" Carlos asks.

So this is all about the shower I gave her tonight, I think to myself.

"We alternate," I reply. "Sometimes I do it. Sometimes Susan does it."

He nods, never looking up at me, writing furiously.

"What would you say is the percentage of the time you wash her?"

"Fifty. Susan and I split everything with Janni. We've always done everything fifty-fifty."

Carlos nods, still writing. "When you wash her, do you wash her privates?"

"Yes."

"Has she ever complained of pain or discomfort when you wash her genitals, and did she ever ask you to stop?"

I sigh. This is going to make me look bad, but I have to tell the truth.

"Yes," I say. "Once when I was washing her vagina she complained that I was too rough."

He looks up. "And what happened?"

"I apologized and stopped."

"And when was this?"

"Last summer sometime."

He goes back to his notepad.

"Anything else?"

"Not that I am aware of."

He nods. "Okay." He looks up from the clipboard. "Well, you are correct. I am here because a claim of sexual abuse has been made against you." He exhales and shifts his feet, uncomfortably. "The claim is that you inserted your finger into her vagina."

Nausea sweeps over me. For some reason, I wasn't prepared for him to be so graphic. The thought of that happening to any little girl is horrendous, but the thought of it happening to Janni is more than I can bear.

I bend over, afraid I might puke.

"Are you okay?" I hear Carlos ask. Again, he sounds strangely sincere.

I can't speak.

"Do you need a minute?" Carlos asks.

I come back to my full height, sucking in air like I'm hyperventilating. "No. Let's get through this."

"You sure you're going to be okay?"

"Please," I pant. "Just do what you gotta do."

He nods. "Okay. I hate to ask this, but the law requires that I do: Did you ever insert your finger into January's vagina?"

Another wave of nausea.

"Not intentionally," I manage.

"What do you mean, 'not intentionally'?"

"If she said I did that, then it must have been an accident while I was washing her, like that time I told you."

"Is there any other reason you can think of that would cause her to say something like that?"

I feel hot. Blood is pounding through my body. "No," I say forlornly. The fact that she believes I hurt her like that is worse than anything else.

He looks up at me, then pauses as I wait for him to tell the deputy to arrest me, but instead he returns to his clipboard.

"Well, she didn't actually say that."

I stare at him.

"What?" is all I can manage.

He lowers the clipboard. "I've already been out to interview Janni. I did that before I came here. She didn't corroborate the claim. She said exactly what you said . . ." He flips back in his notes. " 'Fifty percent of the time Mommy washes me and fifty percent of the time Daddy washes me.' "

"She . . . She didn't say . . . that?" I can't bring myself to repeat it.

Carlos shakes his head. "Nope."

"Then why . . . why did you say that?"

"Because that was what the person who called in the report said she said."

"Who?"

Carlos shakes his head. "I can't tell you. Those who report child abuse are protected by confidentiality laws."

"So what happens now?" I ask.

"Well, since she is not currently in the home, she is not in any immediate danger. All we ask is that you cooperate with our investigation and the hospital's rules. They have asked that you not give Janni showers anymore while she is there. Not just you. Your wife as well."

He hands me a sheet on his clipboard. "This gives our office permission to have Janni sent to a forensic pathologist for examination. This is a pretty standard thing. It's just something we have to do before we can close our investigation."

I slowly reach for the clipboard and pen he is holding out to me. "That's it?"

He nods. "That's it."

I sign the document and Carlos extends his hand. "Thank you very much, Mr. Schofield, and sorry to bother you so late." He moves to the door, forcing the hulking deputy to step aside.

"We're done?" the deputy asks, unfolding his arms, looking surprised.

"We're done," Carlos replies. "Let's go."

The deputy seems disappointed.

"SHOULD I STILL visit Janni?" I ask Carlos. We're all sitting around the kitchen table signing the necessary documents for the investigation to move forward.

"I think you should keep doing what you've been doing," he answers. "As long as you follow the guidelines of the hospital. Besides, I think she needs to see her father. If you don't come, she isn't going to understand why."

"So you don't think I actually did this?" I ask him.

He doesn't answer right away, then says, "What I think doesn't matter."

I nod, understanding.

"But," he suddenly adds, "for what it's worth . . ." He looks me in the eye. "No, I don't."

THE NEXT NIGHT at visiting hours, I come in with Susan and Bodhi. Nurse Ratched looks shocked to see me. I wonder if she was the one who called DCFS on me, but I decide to follow Carlos's advice and let it go. Besides, Janni's awake this time.

"Hey, sweetie," I call to her, unsure how she'll react to me after all this investigation.

But she doesn't react differently at all. In fact, she's calmer than usual.

"Did you bring food?" she asks, simply.

"Ahhh," I wince, preparing for her to scream or hit me.

"We forgot." Susan immediately apologizes. "But we'll bring whatever you want tomorrow."

Janni thinks for a moment. "Del Taco," she finally says.

I am shocked. She didn't blow up.

"Have you had anything to eat today?" Susan asks.

"I ate a grilled cheese," Janni replies.

Susan and I exchange looks.

"So no PRNs today?" Susan asks.

"I got a Thorazine injection," she says as though she just got some candy.

Susan and I look at each other again.

"When?" I ask.

Janni shrugs. "Sometime today."

"Why?" Susan asks.

Janni shrugs again. "I couldn't stop hitting, so I asked for one so I wouldn't hit."

I can't believe what I am hearing.

"You asked for it?" Susan repeats the question, clearly unable to believe it, either.

Janni nods. "It helps me calm down."

I get up and go to the nurses' station and call over Nurse Ratched. "Did Janni get a Thorazine injection today?"

"I don't think so," she answers, clearly not wanting to talk to me.

"Can you check the logbook?"

She disappears. A few minutes later she returns. "I was wrong. She got two."

"Two?"

"She got the first one because she was being abusive to staff. Then about two hours later she came up and said she needed another."

I turn away, stunned. Janni has had a double shot of Thorazine today and is still awake. Not only is she still awake, she is calmer than I can remember her being. Ever.

CHAPTER SEVENTEEN

April 5, 2008

Every morning I walk from the parking lot to my classroom and begin the process of pushing all my emotions down. By the time I open the door and say good morning to my students, the process is almost complete. I sit down at the desk in front of the room and take out my materials. I only have fifty minutes of class time, but I can't start immediately. I have to sit there for a few minutes, silent, because I am still thinking about what is happening to Janni and I can't teach in that state of mind.

I look down at the assignments they turned in last week that I haven't responded to. I can't look up at my students, not yet. I can't because right now I despise them. I hate them because they have no idea what I'm going through. I hate them because even if I tried to explain it they wouldn't understand. They're eighteen years old. I was eighteen once. It wasn't that long ago, but it may as well have been another life. But mostly I hate them because they are here out of hope. I don't feel any hope anymore, and I envy them for that. And envy turns to hate.

I hear my students clearing their throats, waiting for me. I get up and pace between the walls of the classroom. I stop in front of the class. The transformation is complete. I am no longer Janni's father and Susan's husband. I turn and look at them for the first time.

"Okay," I say, a smile on my face, ready to teach. Suddenly, I am animated and entertaining, cracking jokes to get my students engaged. And they never know.

Once class is over, Professor Schofield has no one to perform for. Alone, in my office, Janni's father begins to creep back in, chipping away at Professor Schofield. I fight him off. I still have work to do.

My cell rings. It's Susan. I open my phone, instantly shifting into the role of Susan's husband. "Doe?" I answer, still using my pet name for her out of habit. I can hear the sound of windblast in the background. Susan is on the road.

"I'm taking Janni to UCLA."

"What happened?" I ask, my voice flat. Susan's husband doesn't feel. He can't afford to feel. I know something has happened, but it can't be about Janni and Bodhi because Bodhi is still safely with Jeanne. Whatever has happened, Susan is just freaking out and now my job is to talk her down off the ledge.

"She went crazy at the bagel place in Burbank this morning. We were going to the zoo for a playdate, but I had to cancel. She ran behind the counter and started pulling things out and throwing them on the floor. I had to get the employees there to help me get her out. I told them, 'I'm sorry. My daughter has schizophrenia.'"

I sigh. "She doesn't have schizophrenia."

"Then what is it!?" Susan shouts at me. "Huh? Do you know? It took all these employees to help me get Thorazine into her, and that was already her second dose of the day!"

"She's only been out of Alhambra for four days," I reply calmly.

I feel like Susan is giving up too quickly. "They said there would be an adjustment period." In truth, I don't want her to go back, even to UCLA. Not yet. When she came home from Alhambra, she came home to a new apartment, a two-bedroom in the same complex. We had moved while she was gone. I proudly presented her with her very own room, decorated in a rainbow theme just like she'd told us she wanted. My father had even come out to help me set it up.

"I don't care what Alhambra said," Susan retorts. "She needs to go back to the hospital."

"How is she right now?" I ask.

"She's asleep. The Thorazine finally kicked in."

I breathe a sigh of relief. "Why don't you just go home? I'll leave now and meet you there."

"*No.* I'm taking her to UCLA. You can pick up Bodhi and go home if you like. You don't need to come. I did this on my own last time and I can do it again."

It is the forcefulness of the "no" that shocks me. Our marriage has always been one of equals. We've always talked and made sure we agreed. Now Susan is making decisions regarding Janni without any consideration of how I feel.

"What if they don't have any beds?" I reply, keeping my voice even. "She's asleep. She'll stay asleep until I get home. It's over now. Just go home."

"No," Susan says again, even more defiantly.

"Why?" I cry.

"Because you will go to work tomorrow and I will be left to deal with Janni on my own. I can't do it. She needs UCLA. Like I said, you don't have to come. Just pick up Bodhi."

The "you don't have to come" makes my blood boil. It feels like she's implying I'm not needed. I can check out.

"I'm coming."

"You don't have to," she challenges me.

"I will get Bodhi and come meet you."

I hang up the phone and stand, collecting my things. Something is wrong. The first time Susan took Janni to the hospital, I believed that I could have kept Janni out. I felt guilt and anger. But this time, I feel terror, because whatever is going on with Janni is beyond my ability to fix. Terror, however, is not a useful emotion for getting things done. Janni's father gets things done. He takes care of problems. He has a job to do. He has to get his family through the day. That is his only goal.

WHEN I GET to the UCLA ER, I discover Janni running down the corridor, completely naked, nurses trying to corral her back into the exam room. She took off her clothes and was trying to run out of the ER.

Susan's just sitting in a chair in the exam room, looking exhausted. I'm stunned by her lack of action.

"She's running naked in the hall!" I say to her.

"I know. She spilled water on herself, freaked out, and took all of her clothes off. They offered her a gown, but she refuses to wear it."

"She can't run naked in the hall!"

"I know that," Susan replies as if I am the biggest idiot in the world, "but she won't listen to me and nobody will help."

"We need to at least get her into the room."

Susan shakes her head. "I'm done. I'm tired of doing this alone. Let her run naked through the halls. They need to see what we deal with every day. Then maybe they'll get off their asses and get a psychiatrist down here."

"She still hasn't gotten a psych consult?" I ask incredulously. They've already been here for four hours.

"Nope," Susan replies. "I guess they don't take us seriously enough. I guess she has to run naked through the halls and mess up their computer systems before they take this seriously."

As angry as I am because a psychiatrist still hasn't come, I'm even angrier with Susan. It's like she's giving up. I put Bodhi's car seat down and run out of the room to chase down Janni. I am not going to let her get hurt. She is punching buttons on a heart monitor when I reach her, thankfully not attached to anyone.

"Janni, you need to come back to the room."

She turns to me, smiles, then returns to punching the buttons. I grab her by her arm and start back to her assigned room. Janni goes to the floor, forcing me to pull her entire weight, which I'm not going to do to her naked over a hard surface.

"Janni, you need to get up. Hospital floors are filthy. You don't know what is on them."

Instead of getting up, she lifts her legs and bicycles them into my stomach, hard.

A nurse comes up. "She can't be out here. She needs to stay in her room."

I go down to the floor and scoop her entire body up in my arms, staggering to my feet under her weight.

"What do you think I'm trying to do?" I grunt at the moronic nurse while Janni punches the sides of my head.

I carry Janni back to her room and put her on the bed. "Janni, you need to put on clothes," I gasp, already exhausted. As soon as I let her go, she bolts for the door again. I grab her, holding her back, while I'm being kicked in the shins and punched in my arms and stomach.

"Let her go," Susan orders me. "This is a hospital. They should be helping. I guess it has to get worse before they'll do something."

I've had it with Susan. "You don't get it, do you?"

"I get it. They don't."

I turn on Susan, still shielding myself from Janni while holding her at the same time.

"What do you think is going to happen if we let her run amok?"

Susan leans forward as if I am too dense to understand her. "Why do they think we are here? Hello?"

I grunt from the pain of being kicked. "Right now what it looks like to them is a mother who makes no effort to control her child."

"I can't control her!" Susan fires back.

"If we just let her go, you know what they'll do? They'll call the cops."

"So? Let them. Maybe then we'll finally get some help."

I lean closer to her and snarl, "I'm being investigated for frickin' molesting my daughter! If the cops get called and they come here and find her running naked and out of control, who are they going to blame?"

"The hospital," Susan replies.

"Us! They will take her away from us! You don't seem to realize that! They will take her into state care because obviously we are unfit to be parents."

"Then what are we supposed to do?"

"Deal with it!"

"I am tired of being hit and having things thrown at me all day long," Susan fires back.

I turn away, trying to control my anger, then back to her. "Just take Bodhi and go home. I will stay with her."

"No. I don't trust you to stay here. You'll leave and bring her home. Nothing will change."

I stare at her. She's right. That is exactly what I will do.

"Nothing is going to change anyway," I finally say.

. . .

AFTER A COUPLE more hours Janni gets her psych consult and they tell us they're going to admit her. My anger at Susan starts to abate. She was right. I didn't have the courage to follow through, but we've finally gotten Janni into UCLA.

Then the attending psychiatrist comes back to tell us they can't admit her.

I stare at her, already starting to lose it. Like Susan, I am tired of being jerked around.

"There are two large teenage boys on the unit right now with anger issues," the psychiatrist tells us. "We can't admit her, because we wouldn't be able to guarantee her safety. But don't worry. In situations like this we arrange transport to the next-closest facility . . . which is BHC Alhambra."

"No!" Susan and I refuse in unison.

"We've already been to Alhambra," Susan explains. "We had bad experiences there."

The psychiatrist nods.

"I understand. We don't want to send her somewhere you're not comfortable with." The only other psychiatric inpatient unit that accepts children Janni's age and has a bed available is Loma Linda University Hospital, one hundred miles away, in Redlands, California.

CHAPTER EIGHTEEN

April 6, 2008

It's a hundred miles out to visit Janni and a hundred miles back. Visiting is from six to seven, so we make sure to leave by 2 P.M. so we're on time and get the full hour. Loma Linda is run by the Seventh Day Adventists, and they're much stricter than Alhambra. They don't allow any outside food. We tried to tell them that Janni will only eat certain foods and we're afraid she'll lose weight, but Barb, the social worker, assures us Janni will be fine. Once again, there are no calls from any doctor. Nor can I get one on the phone.

But at least Loma Linda has separate wings and programs for teens and kids. I can relax, knowing that Janni is safe here.

When we arrive, we have to wait for Janni to be brought out to us in the visiting room, which has toys, books, and puzzles.

Janni enters the room, Barb following. Susan and I stand up.

"Hey, sweetie, how are you?" we both ask.

"I'm fine," Janni answers. "Bodhi!" she exclaims, spotting him in his car seat. I tense, ready to intercede, but she just goes down on her knees next to him. "Baby. I missed you."

She missed him? I am shocked.

"How is she doing?" Susan asks Barb.

"She's doing fine," Barb answers. "She's definitely a strong-willed child. She only wants to do what she wants to do, and sometimes she has to go into the 'time-out' room."

"Is she getting Thorazine?" Susan asks.

"We don't use Thorazine here," Barb replies. "I know some hospitals do, but we don't."

"But it works really well for her," Susan presses. "It helps with the violence."

Barb smiles. "We don't believe in using Thorazine. We use Seroquel as a PRN." Seroquel is another antipsychotic, what is called an "atypical," one of the new classes of antipsychotics developed in the last few years.

"But she's already taking Seroquel," Susan answers her.

"You only have an hour. Why don't you spend it with her," Barb suggests, walking off.

Susan gives me a look of concern. "I don't like that she isn't getting any Thorazine."

"I know, but she just said she missed Bodhi."

Janni rubs her hands. "I love Bodhi."

Is this the same child?

"I thought you hated his crying," I say.

"I do hate his crying," Janni replies.

I spot a box of Legos. "Legos!" I say to Janni. "I loved these as a kid. Janni, do you want to build a house?"

Janni looks at the Legos, deciding if she wants to play, then comes over. I feel a surge of hope. First she missed Bodhi and now she's actually engaging in play.

"What are you eating here?" Susan asks her.

"Toast and butter," Janni answers.

"Anything else?" Susan asks, clearly concerned.

"No."

Susan looks at me, irritated. "I told them she wouldn't eat."

All I care about is getting through this visit and it being a good one. Every good visit means maybe we're getting out of whatever brought this on in the first place. I don't want Susan to rock the boat.

"She's not gonna starve," I say.

"The rats don't like Bodhi," Janni suddenly announces without looking up from the Legos. "My seven rats. They're scared of the big baby."

"They don't have to be scared of Bodhi," I say. "Bodhi won't hurt them. Can you tell them that Bodhi won't hurt them?"

"I do."

"And what do they say?" I ask.

Janni is trying to fit a block on the house I am building. "They won't listen to me."

"Janni, they will listen if you tell them to listen."

She struggles to get a block on and throws it, then knocks over the box of Legos.

"Janni! Why did you do that? Come here and help me clean them up."

"No."

"So, Janni," Susan asks, "how are the other girls here?"

"Fine."

"Do you like any of them?"

"No."

"Are they nice to you?"

"Yes, but I don't like them."

"Why not?"

"Janni, look!" I call, holding up my half-finished Lego house, trying to get her attention back.

"Do they have imaginations like you?" Susan persists.

"No," Janni answers.

I give an exasperated sigh and glare at Susan. I know she doesn't mean to, but I fear that all she is doing is reminding Janni of her differences from everybody else.

Janni moves over to Susan. She looks like she is going in for a hug, so I am not prepared when Janni raises her fist and hits Susan on the arm.

"Janni, no," Susan says, but Janni keeps hitting.

Susan tries to take hold of Janni's arms. "She needs Thorazine," she says to me.

I step out to the nurses' station. "Where's Barb? Janni just hit Susan out of nowhere," I say. "I don't think the meds she's on are enough."

Barb comes around from the nurses' station and enters the visiting room.

I follow, expecting that she wants to see for herself.

"Janni, did you just hit your mother?"

"Yes," Janni answers without emotion.

Barb sighs. "Janni, you know the rules. There is no hitting. If you hit, you lose your visiting privileges." She takes Janni by the hand and Janni screams.

Barb pulls harder, and another nurse joins her as Janni drops to the floor. "Janni, come on."

To my immense shock they drag Janni out of the room. Every parental instinct urges me to leap forward and tell Barb to get her fat hands off my daughter.

"We don't want her to leave," I cry out. "I just wanted you to know the meds aren't working."

"Janni knows the rules," Barb says through gritted teeth as she continues to drag the screaming and hitting Janni through the hallway. "Janni, we have to go to the 'time-out' room."

"She can't control it," Susan cries. "That's why she's here."

"Janni knows that behavior is not acceptable, don't you, Janni?" Barb says.

Janni is still kicking and screaming, like she's fighting for her life. And I, her father, am letting it happen.

"You need to leave now," Barb tells us.

"We'll wait," Susan answers.

"She's not coming back out. Visitation is over for her."

"We drove a hundred miles to see her and we only get an hour!" Susan pleads.

Barb is unmoved. "She needs to learn there are consequences to her actions."

"She needs more medication. She needs Thorazine!" Susan cries. But Bodhi starts to cry and Susan has to turn to him.

I see Barb reach for her keycard to open the time-out room.

"I love you, Janni," I say weakly, but Janni doesn't see me as the nurse tosses her down on the rubber mat. As Janni gets up to take another swing, Barb quickly slams the door, and it locks, leaving Janni screaming inside.

WE ARE SHOCKED when Barb calls to tell us they're planning to discharge Janni on Thursday, only five days after she went in.

Immediately, the overwhelming and crippling sense of fear returns. She's not ready. The violence still explodes out of nowhere. She's still a threat to Bodhi. I've been waiting for a clear sign from Janni that she is better. I want to look into her eyes and feel like the violence is gone for good. But it isn't. Whatever brought on the violence in the first place is still there. Even if Bodhi was the trigger, he is here to stay. We have done everything, to the point that Janni barely knows he exists. Jesus Christ, we barely let him make a sound if we can help it. We have gone as far as we can go in limiting his impact on Janni.

But in my heart of hearts I know it isn't Bodhi. He may have been the final tipping point, but Janni has been changing before my eyes for years. I just didn't want to admit it to myself.

And now Loma Linda is releasing her because they consider her stable enough to go home? They want us to pick her up earlier in the day, but we refuse, demanding to see the doctor. The doctor only sees parents on Thursdays during visiting hours.

"But she's still violent!" Susan cries as we wait in Barb's office for the doctor. "Nothing has changed. You haven't even changed her medications."

"Will it be perfect?" Barb says to us. "No, of course not. January is not an easy child."

"But she is still a threat to Bodhi! How am I supposed to keep him safe?"

"You are going to have to just bite the bullet and be tougher with her," Barb insists.

"I'd like to see you handle her with an *infant* in your arms!" Susan shoots back.

"Look," Barb replies in a way that is meant to be soothing but comes off as condescending, "I raised children and had a very strong-willed child, too. Nobody ever said parenting was easy."

"We never expected it to be 'easy,'" Susan fires back, frustrated. "But we shouldn't have to worry about her hurting Bodhi! We can't live like this!"

Barb nods. "I think I hear the doctor outside. Let me bring him in to talk to you."

She leaves, closing the door behind her.

Barb comes back in with the doctor, who looks like he just got back from shooting eighteen holes of golf. He's tanned, wearing the kind of hideous plaid golfer pants that my grandfather used to wear when he was alive. He sits on the edge of Barb's desk.

"I heard you wanted to see me?" he asks.

"Yes." Susan launches into it. "You've made no med changes. In fact, you've done nothing at all and you're releasing Janni."

"I didn't feel she needed any med changes," he says and smiles. "In fact, I'm convinced that in six months she won't be on any medication at all."

I feel an immense sense of relief. He seems so sure of himself.

"What about schizophrenia?" Susan demands of him.

"I don't see any evidence of schizophrenia. She engages with the nursing staff."

"What about her violence?" She strikes back at him. "It's still there. Does she have to kill Bodhi before you people will do anything?"

"Susan," I say gently. I'm getting tired of her yelling at everyone. Or maybe I am just getting tired of the fight.

She turns on me. "You keep thinking they care, but they don't. If she kills Bodhi, they'll just say 'How tragic' and move on!"

"That's not true," Barb replies. "We care very much."

"Let me ask you a question," the doctor says to Susan. "She was at Alhambra for three weeks, right?"

Susan nods. "And they didn't do a damn thing, either."

The doctor nods understandingly, like he's the doctor out of that famous Norman Rockwell painting. "And how long was she out before you brought her to UCLA?"

"Four days," Susan answers.

The doctor sits back with a knowing look on his face. "So she was only out four days before you took her back to the hospital. What does that tell you?"

"It tells me she still isn't any better, that maybe she has schizophrenia, but nobody will listen to her because of her age. I keep telling her to tell doctors the truth. She says she is telling you, but that you don't believe her!"

"Why are you so convinced she has schizophrenia?" he asks.

"Because the only thing that stops her violence is Thorazine," Susan answers.

"Thorazine is a sedative. It would stop anybody's violence."

"That's not true. Janni has been on antipsychotics before and they did nothing. She ran around like she was on nothing at all," Susan retorts.

I don't know why I'm not speaking up and am letting Susan do all the arguing. Maybe I'm tired of the uncertainty. I'm tired of living in fear. I'm tired of nobody being able to fix this.

"I can't speak to that," the doctor responds, "but don't you think four days is a pretty short time to be out in the world before bringing her back to the hospital?"

"We couldn't handle her! She was out of control."

The doctor softens his tone. "You know what my diagnosis of Janni is? Severe anxiety." He sighs, like he's trying to make us understand a difficult concept that we aren't getting. "As adults, we forget what it's like to be a kid. The world is a pretty scary place."

"We're scared of Janni harming her brother!" Susan says, exasperated.

"You said she was in Alhambra for three weeks and she liked it. She didn't want to leave. Then she gets out, has a bad day, as kids do, as we all do, and you bring her straight back to the hospital," the doctor says. "You know what that is teaching her?"

Susan stares at him, angrily waiting for his answer.

"It's teaching her that when life gets too hard, run away. That's why I think we don't see the level of violence you describe here, although I don't doubt it happens at home. She even likes it here. She's told Barb and all the staff she likes it here."

"Because she is with other kids who are like her," Susan retorts.

The doctor shakes his head. "No, she likes it here because she doesn't have to deal with problems in her world, like her feelings for

Bodhi. I don't doubt you care about her. You are both obviously very committed parents. But every time you bring her back to the hospital, all you're doing is giving her a way of not dealing with life. That is how people become institutionalized. I used to see it when the state hospitals were around, and it was the same thing. It's not like what you see in the movies. Most patients didn't want to leave. They didn't want to leave because life was easier on the inside."

"She can't control it," Susan insists. "She says she can't control it."

The doctor shrugs. "Seems like she can control it when she wants to. The question is do the two of you ever actually ask her to control it or do you just accept that there is something wrong and there is nothing you can do about it?"

"We've been working with her since the day she was born!" Susan is nearly out of breath from yelling. "She was always different. She never slept as a baby. We had to take her out all day, every day, to get her enough stimulation so she would sleep a little. Even when she was sick, it didn't slow her down at all. We still had to take her out."

"Will you let the man speak?" I finally interject. "Getting angry isn't going to solve anything."

"They're not doing anything!" Susan retorts. "They don't listen to her."

"How many times are we going to keep bringing her back to the hospital and get the same answer?" I demand. "Has it occurred to you that maybe we keep getting the same answer because maybe they are right?"

"Fine," Susan says. "You believe these idiots if you want to."

I wince. I know she is as frustrated as I am, but I hate it when she attacks the doctors so openly.

"So what do you propose we do?" I ask the doctor.

"Stand up to her," he says simply.

"She doesn't take no for an answer," Susan says with hostility.

"She will eventually," the doctor replies. "It is going to be tough, I won't lie to you, but you have to stand up and hold your ground. Right now all she sees in you two is fear, and that creates fear in her. That is why she is lashing out. Stop being afraid and she will stop lashing out."

"He's right," I say.

Susan glares at me. "What do you mean, 'He's right'?"

"We live in constant fear of her."

"We live in fear because she tries to hurt Bodhi!"

"But she never actually has."

"Because we stop her." Susan is condescending.

"But we are the parents!" I say, pounding my chest. "We shouldn't be living in fear of our own child!"

The doctor gently interjects. "I'm telling you, you need to get tougher on her. It's going to be damn hard in the beginning, because you're going to have to be tough with every infraction. Don't give an inch. Let her know that her behavior is unacceptable."

"We've tried that!" Susan shouts.

"No, we haven't," I answer her. "As soon as the violence started, we ran straight to a shrink. We never stood up to her."

"You're the one who is always giving in to her, just to keep the peace!"

"I was wrong."

"Why are you so cocky all of a sudden?"

I don't really know. Maybe it is because doctors keep telling me nothing is wrong with Janni, so Susan is the only other target I have. "I'm sick of being the one who does everything to keep this family going!"

"You don't do everything! Who takes Janni so you can work?"

"And what do you do? Call me at work constantly, saying how you can't handle it!"

Susan gives me a disgusted look, like I'm a worm. "You're just perfect, aren't you?"

The doctor reaches out and puts one hand on Susan's shoulder and one on mine. "See what she is doing to both of you? She's destroying your family. And letting her do it is not going to help any of you, most especially her. If you don't stand up to her now, this will only get worse."

He's right. We've been living in fear and I'm tired of it. Janni is already headed down the path to being a juvenile delinquent. Everything she could be, all her potential, will be lost, and I will not let that happen. If I have to be the parent I never wanted to be, the ballbusting father who gives no quarter, I will do it. I will not let Janni throw her life away.

ONCE JANNI IS handed over to us, there is no more time for fighting. The focus is back to Janni. The simmering anger between Susan and me must be pushed down.

After completing the discharge from Loma Linda, we go to the nearby Red Lobster to celebrate Janni's homecoming. Not that it feels anything like a celebration; rather it feels like trying to eat in the trenches of World War I, never knowing when the shelling is going to start again.

Susan sits across from me. Bodhi, in his car seat, sits in a sling at the edge of the table. Janni chooses to sit next to me like she usually does, although "sitting" is a stretch. She is bouncing around, standing up on the booth seat to look for her food. Every time I tell her to get down, she does, only to pick up an object like the saltshaker, preparing to throw it.

"Janni, if you throw that, we are leaving right now," I say, already trying to make the transition to "tough parent," which doesn't come easy to me. What I really want is to have a nice, peaceful dinner. Usually, in restaurants, I have to work constantly to engage her in something while we wait for the food, but not tonight. Tonight she's going to have to wait.

Janni looks at me, trying to decide if I am serious. I give her a look that I am and she puts the saltshaker down. "But I'm hungry!"

"That's no excuse for throwing something," I reply.

"But I'm hungry," Janni says again, as if this explains it. "The food is taking soooo long!"

The fact that the waitress only took our order five minutes ago and that a certain amount of time is needed to prepare it means nothing to Janni.

"Then have a biscuit." I offer her one.

"No."

"Then you aren't that hungry."

"I was a picky eater," Susan says.

I glare at her. She's not helping. If this is going to work, we need to be a united front. Janni can't think one parent will give in when the other won't. These are actually the first words Susan has spoken to me since we left Loma Linda.

The waitress brings cheese sticks and Janni grabs one.

"They're going to be hot," I tell Janni.

Janni ignores me, takes a bite, and then immediately opens her mouth and lets the half-chewed cheese stick fall from her mouth onto the floor under the booth.

"Hot!" Janni complains.

I sigh irritably. "I told you they'd be hot. You need to give them a few minutes to cool."

Instead of waiting, Janni picks up another cheese stick, bites into it, and spits the pieces back out.

"Janni, I said to wait!"

"But I'm hungry!" she whines.

"What good is trying to eat them if they're too hot? Just give them a minute to cool."

Janni picks up yet another cheese stick, puts it in her mouth, complains it's too hot, and spits it out.

"Janni," I say, exasperated by her inability to wait for anything. "You're wasting them!"

Janni abruptly slips underneath the booth and down onto the floor.

"Janni, what are you doing?" I demand.

"Will you stop yelling at her?" Susan complains. "She just got out of the hospital."

I lean over to see what Janni is doing under the table. She is crouched down over the floor, picking up the spit-out pieces of cheese stick, shoving them into her mouth like a rat.

"Janni, don't eat off the floor!" My voice rises, but she ignores me. It's an unnerving sight, not like when toddlers pick candy up off the ground, but like someone so starving they're rummaging through scraps of food fallen from the table.

"Janni, there are plenty of cheese sticks still on the plate," I say, trying to reason with her.

"Let it go," Susan says to me.

I look up at her, stunned. "I'm not going to let her eat off the floor! It's not right!"

"Since when do you care about social etiquette?" Susan asks, choosing this moment to get in another shot at me.

But this is different. Janni looks inhuman. Now she's not even using her hands, simply putting her head down and eating off the floor with her mouth. She's regressing, not getting better.

"Janni, get up here or we're leaving."

She ignores me.

I reach down and grab her, pulling her up. I'm not going to let my daughter turn into an animal.

"Careful!" Susan warns. "Watch her head."

Janni scurries farther under the table, out of my reach. Swearing under my breath, I go down underneath the booth and grab her legs, pulling. She screams, an earsplitting scream that makes the entire restaurant look our way.

"Okay, that's it. Come on, Janni."

"Where are we going?"

"We're going for a time-out."

"We're not at home," Janni answers smugly. "There's nowhere to give me a time-out."

"We're going to the car," I reply, sliding back out from under the table, pulling Janni with me, nearly knocking over Bodhi's car seat sling in the process.

Janni comes up screaming and hitting me. I can't see, but I feel the other restaurant patrons staring at my back.

"We're going to wait in the car until you decide you're ready to behave."

"But I'm hungry," Janni cries.

"You have to earn the right to come back in," I reply.

Janni wails, pulling against me. I know she'll never just walk out of here with me. I have no choice but to lift her off her feet and sling her over my shoulder like a sack of potatoes. I carry my screaming daughter through the restaurant, ignoring her hitting the back of my head.

When we reach the exit, the hostess looks up to see what the commotion is, and shock comes over her face.

"Is everything okay?" she asks, standing there stupidly.

"Can you open the door?" I ask angrily.

The hostess snaps out of her shock and runs to open the door. I carry Janni through it, trying to make sure her head doesn't hit the door on the way out, and then we are outside.

It is dark when we reach the car. I'm going to have to put her down to get my car keys out. I do, and immediately she tries to run back into the restaurant, but reflexively my arm shoots out and grabs her. I feel the pinching tug on the tendons in my arm, like a fishing line going tight. Janni comes flying back into me.

I unlock the car, open the passenger door, and push Janni inside, then close the door quickly so she can't get her fingers around the door's frame. I'm not fast enough to get the door completely closed before Janni is pushing against it from the inside. My force against hers, and scarily, they seem equal. She pushes against the door with all her might, while I slam my body into the door and click the lock button on my key.

Janni is screaming, not her usual scream when something doesn't go her way, but a continuous scream, like death itself is in the car with her. But I have no time to think. Janni is smart enough to know how to unlock the door. She presses the button unlocking all the doors and the passenger door swings opens.

My left arm pushes the door closed while my right hand presses the lock button. She turns from me, jumping across the gearshift in the center console to the driver's side. I race around the front of the car and throw my body into the driver's-side door as it opens, hitting the lock button again.

She tries again, but I hold the door closed.

"I need to get out!" she screams at me, throwing her hands against the window, the heat radiating out and fogging up the glass.

"Not until you calm down." I'm not angry. She just has to know that she's not going to win.

She climbs over the center console into the backseat, headed for the driver's-side rear door, but I get there first and push my hand against it, keeping her from opening the door. Janni turns and stumbles across the backseat, tripping over Bodhi's car seat base, to the passenger side. Seeing her going, I race over to the other side of the car so I can keep the passenger-side rear door closed. In the back of my mind, it registers how insane this is, like a twisted game of Whack-A-Mole. Whatever door she moves toward to try to escape, I get there first to keep that door closed.

"When you calm down and tell me you are ready to behave, I will let you out," I say calmly through the glass. "This is not a punishment. This is only until you calm down."

Janni launches herself over the backseat and into the rear area of our small SUV. I move to the back of the car, watching for any sign that she's calming down so I can let her out. She pounds on the rear window, so hard that it must hurt her hands.

"Janni, don't do that!" I call in through the window. "You could break your hands!" I know I am the one doing this to her, but all we've gone through has to end somewhere.

"Let me out!" she screams. "Please!"

"Not until you calm down," I repeat, trying very hard to keep my voice even.

Janni turns away from me, looking around. We have sand toys back there from the days when we used to go to the park. She picks up a bucket and throws it against the glass. It bounces harmlessly off.

She searches frantically through the toys, repeatedly hurling them against the glass. *Just give in, Janni. I know the world is too stupid for you. I'm sorry, but continuing on this path is not going to make the world see your genius. It is just going to get you locked up.*

Having run out of items to throw, she climbs over to the front seat and picks up her CD case, smashing it against the windshield.

"Janni, if you break those, I'm not buying new ones. I don't care if you destroy the car. I'm not letting you out until you calm down." *You won't win, Janni. Better I break you than the world breaks you.*

Finally, she throws herself against the driver's-side window, tears streaming down her cheeks and a terrified look on her face. Every instinct makes me want to let her out. I don't know if this is the right thing to do or not. I wish some expert were here to reassure me I'm doing the right thing.

"Take me back!" she wails.

"Take you back where?"

"To the hospital!"

To the hospital. She wants to run back to the hospital. She actually prefers it to the world out here. This world terrifies her.

I have to get her through this fear.

"No," I answer. I can't bear to see her like this. Violence I can deal with, not terror. She looks like a child now. But I have to see this through. I might be the only one left who can save her. I harden my heart. "We are not going back to the hospital."

"I need to go back! Just let me go back!"

She is like a cornered animal. I look away. *You've got to do this, Michael. Otherwise she will become institutionalized. She didn't want to leave Alhambra. Loma Linda is right. She has got to learn to deal with life.*

I look back. "We're not going back to the hospital, Janni!"

"Please! I need to go back!"

"I'm not taking you back."

"I want to go back!"

"No."

She turns from the window and sits on her knees in the driver's seat, sobbing.

I sigh, leaning against the car door, exhausted, looking in at her. Maybe we've finally turned a corner. She came at me with her worst violence and I stood my ground.

"It's gonna be okay, Janni," I say through the glass. "We'll get through this."

CHAPTER NINETEEN

May 2008

The door to Janni's bedroom has a lock on it, as most bedroom doors do, designed to protect the privacy of the occupant.

I get a Phillips-head screwdriver out of my tool kit and unscrew the door handles on both the inside and outside. Then I turn the handles around, putting the handle with the lock on the outside of the door.

If Janni screams, I no longer yell at her. If she hits, I no longer tell her that is unacceptable. I just order her into her room for a time-out. She never goes willingly, of course, so I have to drag her in.

This morning, I came out of the shower to find Susan, holding Bodhi, running in terror into our bedroom and locking the door, with Janni on the outside smashing her fists into the door. So I grab Janni and drag her to her room, silently cursing Susan for not standing up to a five-year-old child and for the fact that I can't even have five minutes to take a shower or go to the bathroom without everything falling apart while I'm gone. Once Susan hears that I'm back, she comes out of the bedroom, only to tell me to be careful with Janni.

"Don't hurt her!" she cries as I drag Janni by her feet over the carpet. One second she is screaming at me to get out of the shower to come help her because Janni is hitting, and the next moment she is criticizing my response.

Once I get Janni into her room, I tell her to think about what she did and I start to leave. Janni immediately gets to her feet and tries to get to the door before I can close it. I need to get out quickly before Janni can get her hand in to block the door closing. I don't want to slam the door on her hand.

So we wind up locked in a battle at the threshold of her room, her trying to push out past me and me trying to push her back in. Eventually, the only way I can get the door closed is to shove her hard enough that she falls backward onto her bed.

She lands on her bed and sits up, a shocked look on her face like she can't understand why I just did that. I can't take that look. I turn away and close the door.

TONIGHT IS OPEN House Night at Janni's kindergarten, and we are going. I watch Susan in the bathroom, putting on makeup. I can't remember the last time I saw her put on makeup. I pull on my suit jacket, glancing at Susan, who is wearing a nice black dress and heels. Looking at us in the mirror, no one would have any idea what we've just been through over the past five months.

Janni walks in, wearing a black-and-white dress Susan bought for her.

"You look beautiful," Susan says to her.

Janni screams, as she does whenever somebody gives her a compliment.

"Janni," I say firmly. "Enough."

"I need to brush your hair." Susan reaches for a hairbrush and begins trying to detangle Janni's natural curls. Janni screams and pulls away.

"Janni," I warn her. "Do you want a time-out?" My voice is calm, cool, controlled.

"It hurts," Janni whines, trying to pull her head away from Susan's brushing.

"That's because you don't brush it," I answer, flatly. "Either you let Mommy do it or you do it. Your choice." My voice makes it completely clear that those are the only two options.

"I'll do it." Janni takes the brush from Susan and digs into her mass of hair, wrenching it down so hard that strands of hair pull free.

"Gentle," I command. "You don't have to be so rough." Janni is pulling on her hair with far more force than Susan, yet she isn't complaining.

"Smooth strokes," Susan says, trying to help, but Janni pulls away, continuing to rip the brush down her hair.

"Doesn't that hurt?" I ask.

"No," Janni answers simply.

Janni finishes and puts down the brush. I look at our reflection in the mirror. We look like a normal family.

SUSAN PUSHES BODHI'S stroller while I walk behind Janni toward the kindergarten classroom. Since starting kindergarten back in January, Janni has missed more than four weeks of school. Fortunately, she hasn't missed anything she didn't already know.

Inside the classroom, I take the time to say hello to other parents, something I have never done. I shake hands with other fathers and make small talk about what we do for a living.

Janni shows us her desk and her art projects. I make no silly jokes like I used to, instead making the same bland comments I hear the other fathers making. Out of the corner of my eye, I watch other fathers, and I model my behavior after them. They treat their sons and daughters like children. That was my mistake. I always treated Janni like an adult. She is a child, and no matter her genius, she needs a strong parent.

A little girl comes over to Janni. "Hi, Janni," she says.

"Hi," Janni answers, no excitement in her voice.

The little girl, of Asian descent, dances away.

"She seems nice," I say to Janni. "What's her name?"

"Amanda."

"Do you ever play with her?"

"Sometimes."

"Well, why don't you go talk to her? She's got a nice dress on, too. Go over to her and tell her you like her dress." If I have to force social interaction, I will. But Janni complies.

I wander around the classroom, trying to figure out what to do with myself. I'm so used to being Janni's shadow. I feel like I just got out of prison. Everything around me, the classroom, being around other families, feels like a distant memory of another life.

I overhear Susan talking to the teacher, who is commenting on how well Janni has been doing since she came back from Loma Linda.

Out of force of habit, I look around for Janni. I don't see her. I come up to Susan. "Where's Janni?"

Susan turns to the front of the class and points. "She's over there, playing with Amanda."

I follow her gaze. Janni is standing right next to Amanda. Each one has a dry-erase marker and they are drawing pictures on the board, side by side.

"Janni, Janni," I hear Amanda say. "Can you do this?" She starts drawing a picture. Janni follows. I hear laughter. Janni is laughing along with Amanda.

I look to their right, at the "streetlight" system on the whiteboard, my eyes moving left to right, from red to yellow to green. Nobody's name is in red. There are a few names in yellow, but most of the names are in green, including Janni's.

I am proud of Janni, yet nothing in my demeanor changes. I remain flat, calm, and in control. Janni is still on the Seroquel and Depakote, but I don't believe that is why she is doing better. I have laid down the law. I am forcing Janni to deal with the real world.

CHAPTER TWENTY

June 2008

Today is our weekly visit with Dr. Howe.

"I have to admit things are a lot better now," Susan is saying. "We used to have ten to twelve violent incidents a day; now it's down to two or three. It's not perfect, but it's manageable."

Dr. Howe nods and turns to Janni, who is playing with the dollhouse. "Janni, how are things going?"

"Good," Janni answers flatly, not looking up.

"How's school? Are you liking it any better?"

"Yes."

"I hear you have a friend now."

"Magical 61," Janni answers.

"No, Janni," I say, "a real friend."

"She is real."

"Who's Magical 61?" Dr. Howe asks.

"A girl."

"What about Amanda?" Susan presses. "You like Amanda."

"Not as much as I like my other friends."

"Why not?" Dr. Howe asks.

"My other friends never leave."

"Do you think we can maybe start reducing her meds?" Susan asks. "She's still on three hundred milligrams of Seroquel and five hundred milligrams of Depakote."

Dr. Howe nods and turns back to us. "Hmmm, she seems to be doing well for the moment. Let's just leave things as they are."

I don't get this. "But she was on the same doses before she went to Loma Linda and they weren't doing anything. Nothing changed until I started getting stricter with her."

Dr. Howe looks at me out of the corner of her eye. "Sometimes it takes the medicine time to work. If it's not broke, don't fix it."

I think back to our first session with Dr. Howe after Janni was released from Loma Linda. I told her what the Loma Linda doctor had said about expecting that in six months Janni would no longer be on medication.

"Maybe" was all Dr. Howe said back then; she was still cautious in not wanting to lower her dosages.

Now she is happy Janni is doing better but still doesn't want to take her off the medication. It is as if she is still not sure the violent storm that has hung over us for the past six months is really gone. I want to believe, need to believe, that it is finally over.

I SIT ON the couch in the living room, waiting while Susan gives Janni her bath.

I don't give Janni baths anymore. I haven't since she was released from Alhambra.

Over in the side pocket of my briefcase is the letter that arrived today from DCFS. *Our investigation into the claim of sexual abuse is hereby officially closed. The allegations were determined to be unfounded and/or unsubstantiated.*

Unsubstantiated. I don't like that word. I realize this is probably a form letter, but it bothers me because "unsubstantiated" leaves the door open. When this first happened, I was more worried about what would happen to Janni than about what would happen to me. I knew I had nothing to hide. I figured DCFS would do their investigation and eventually it would be over. When the letter arrived, I thought it was finished. Then Susan says, "I should still be the one to keep giving Janni her baths."

I stare at her, not understanding.

"It's just not worth the risk," Susan continues.

"But I didn't do anything."

"I know that, but an accusation was still made against you. Yes, you were cleared, but what if you get accused again? They'll look back over their files and see you were accused once before and why take that risk? There's no need for you to give Janni baths anymore."

"I thought I was being a good father, helping out."

"I know, and you did. But you can't do that anymore. Look, I don't like it, either. It means more work for me. She really needs to bathe herself. Also, you need to make sure you are never alone with any girls."

This annoys me.

"When am I ever alone with any girls other than Janni?"

"I'm just saying that you don't want to put yourself in a position where there will be any question at all."

Now I know. This will never really be over. No matter what the letter says, this will hang over me for the rest of my life.

Susan starts to turn away.

"You cried out."

"What?"

"That night when they came. I heard you cry out from the bed-room. You were so upset Carlos had me hold Bodhi."

"Of course I was upset. I couldn't believe what he was telling me."

"Did you believe him?"

Susan hesitates and I have my answer.

"I didn't know what to believe," she answers. "He was telling me all this stuff like it was fact."

I feel ripped apart. How could she possibly have thought me capable of that, even for a second?

"Did you ask her?" I ask, my voice amazingly level.

"Yes, I did. Wouldn't you have if you were in my position?"

I nod. "Of course. I would be worried if you hadn't asked her." But that's a lie. I am devastated. Susan has known me for thirteen years. I thought she knew me better than that.

CHAPTER TWENTY-ONE

September 2008

After dinner, I go into Janni's bedroom and open her backpack. Her "take-home" folder is thicker than usual. First, there are two or three pages of activities related to the lesson of the day. Then there is a "daily homework" sheet. Each student is expected to do one assignment each from the "reading list," "writing list," and "spelling/vocabulary list." To do everything will take two or three hours of nonstop work. And then there's a small white notepaper clipped to a stack of assignments. It's from her new first-grade teacher, Mrs. Parris. I read it.

Janni refused to do her work in class. I am sending it home for completion, along with her regular homework.

I flip through the papers behind the note from Mrs. Parris. It isn't just the work Janni refused to do in class today. It looks like a whole week's worth of assignments.

I sit down on the floor, feeling overwhelmed. It's eight o'clock at night. Janni is out on the couch, finally getting sleepy from all the Seroquel and Depakote she's had today. There is no way I can get her through even half of this stuff. I exhale, trying to stay calm.

"Come on, Janni. We need to do your homework."

"I'm tired," Janni yells from the living room.

I look at the unfinished work. One page is about identifying nouns and verbs. Janni has known this since before she was two. I remember driving around and quizzing her, and she would get it right every time.

I emerge from Janni's room and go into our bedroom, where Susan is sacked out on the bed.

"It would be helpful if you had her do some homework right after school, when she is not wiped out from the meds."

"When I pick her up, I have to take her out for stimulation. Have you forgotten Janni won't just stay at home? How am I supposed to keep her occupied for five hours until you get home, while protecting Bodhi?"

"Make her do her homework."

"With a baby in my arms?"

"Put Bodhi down and work with her."

"You don't know what I go through with both of them while you're at work. You've forgotten."

"I used to take both of them when you went to work." Susan was just laid off from her job.

"That was only two days! And now I'm constantly on the go with them when Janni is out of school. I take them places where I can keep Janni entertained. I don't come home until right before you do."

I sigh, exasperated. "And then it's on me. You need to be tougher on her."

"I'm exhausted!"

"So am I. I've been teaching all day."

Susan sits up, angry. "It's not the same. You don't have to worry about Janni running off. What am I supposed to do if that happens? Run after her with Bodhi in my arms? Or just leave him?"

"Calmly tell her that if she doesn't come back, you're leaving. If there were consequences, she would eventually get the message. But you don't enforce the rules. You keep taking her places she wants to go because it's easier for you."

"Yes, I do." Susan stares defiantly at me. "I am alone. I do what I have to do to get through the day until you get home." She lies back down. "By the way, it's not like I have the time while she's in school to myself. Every day I take Bodhi and meet Janni at school."

"You shouldn't be going there."

"I have to. The only way Janni will even go to school is if I promise to come meet her for lunch."

This is true. Every morning when I drop Janni off at school, she asks me when Mommy is coming.

"She's got to learn to function in society."

"Mrs. Parris doesn't like her, and Janni senses that."

"No, you don't like Mrs. Parris because she doesn't teach Janni what you think she needs to be learning."

"Yes! She's a genius!"

"Nobody will give a damn unless she learns to follow the rules." I turn away from Susan and go back out into the living room, where Janni is falling asleep on the couch. "Come on, Janni. I know you're tired. Mommy should have had you start your homework earlier, but she didn't."

"I don't want to," Janni mumbles. "I'm too tired."

"Let's just do a little," I reply. "I'll help you."

Janni walks into her room and plunks down at the special desk we got for her.

"I'm tired," she complains again.

"I know. Let's just do three. Which one do you want to do first?"

"This one." She points to a homework sheet with a cat.

"Okay." I read the directions. "Write a paragraph and then circle the nouns. That should be easy." I hand her a pencil.

"What should I say?" she asks.

"Write something about a cat," I reply.

I have a cat named 400. She is an orange tabby. She starts on the "y" in "tabby," but drags the tail of the "y" far down the page, like she can't stop. She reaches the bottom of the page.

"That's not right," she says, more to herself than to me.

"It's okay," I say, handing her an eraser. But Janni takes the eraser, throws it, and tears up the sheet of paper.

"Janni, you'd already finished it! Now we have to do it all over again!" I close my eyes, struggling to stay calm.

"I don't want to." Janni is staring straight ahead at the wall.

I exhale, pushing my hair back. "Janni, you need to do your work." Janni turns to me and hits me on the arm.

"Okay, Janni. Ten-minute time-out for hitting." I start to walk out. Janni dives to the floor, for my ankles, to stop me from getting to the door, but I easily step out of the room and lock the door behind me.

I hear the sound of something heavy hitting the other side of her door. It must be her chair. That is the only large object left in her room that she can pick up and throw. Every time she gets a time-out, she picks up anything she can lift and throws it at the door.

"Now it's fifteen minutes," I call.

She throws the chair again. She's going to break it.

"Twenty minutes," I call out, feeling like a judge increasing the sentence on a prisoner who refuses to cooperate.

I wait, expecting the sound of more items being thrown against the door, but they don't come. I put my ear to the door, trying to hear the scratching sound of pencil on drywall. Typically, once Janni runs out of things to throw, she starts writing on her walls. Things like the word "Lion," the names of her imaginary friends, and phrases that make no sense at all, like "Von Dog."

"Janni," I call through the door. "If you're writing on the walls, you know you'll have to clean it off before coming out of your room." I say this even though it is impossible to get the words off the wall, especially red marker, no matter how hard I scrub.

No answer.

"Janni?"

I unlock the door and open it to find that the room is a mess, with papers strewn everywhere. Her lamp is on the floor.

But no Janni.

"Janni?"

The walk-in closet light is on. I walk over to it and see Janni sitting on the floor, gritting her teeth as she pulls the sleeves of a shirt around her neck.

"What are you doing?" I demand, yanking the shirt away from her. "Don't do that! You'll stretch out your shirts and they won't fit you anymore."

"I want to break my neck," she answers in a voice that is equally dreamy and forceful. She pulls another one of her shirts off a hanger and wraps it around her neck, pulling so hard I can see her hands shaking,

"Janni, stop that!" I grab the second shirt, trying to pull it away, but she clings to it like it's a life preserver.

"Don't do that," I say. My words sound insane even to me. I am commanding her not to try to kill herself?

"I want to know how to break my neck!" Janni screams.

I should ask why in the world she would want to, but I don't. Over the past nine months, our lives have gone to a place I never could have fathomed. I've become numb. Nothing shocks me anymore. It can't. Even this.

"You can't," I simply tell her.

Janni wraps her hands around her neck and squeezes.

"Janni, stop that," I yell, reaching for her hands, trying to get my fingers underneath so I can pull them free.

"What is she doing?" Susan calls, running into the room.

"She says she wants to break her neck," I answer, turning away. I know I should be terrified, but I feel nothing except slight annoyance.

"Oh, my God! Janni!" Susan runs to Janni. "Why do you want to hurt yourself?"

"I want to break my neck."

"You can't, Janni," I say over my shoulder. "It doesn't matter how hard you squeeze. Eventually, you will just pass out and let go." I can't believe how cavalier I sound. Something is seriously wrong with me. Or maybe I'm just tired of always fighting her. But this is my daughter!

"How can I break my neck?" Janni repeats, struggling to keep her hands on her neck.

Susan looks at me. "Help me!"

"She's fine," I say. My voice doesn't sound like my own.

"She's choking herself!" Susan yells at me.

"If she can talk, she can still breathe."

Susan finally manages to pull Janni's hands free. Janni hits at her.

"Why?" Susan asks, tears in her eyes. "Why do you want to break your neck?"

"I don't want to live," Janni replies and goes back to trying to choke herself.

Susan again struggles to get Janni's hands free, then turns to me, her eyes blazing with anger and fear. "She needs to go to the hospital!"

"What's the point?" I reply. "They'll just release her and she'll still be the same."

"Something is wrong!" Susan screams at me. "Can't you see that?"

Yes, but six months ago, I had to stop feeling anything in order to function. Now it appears I can't turn it back on.

"We need to call Dr. Howe! She needs more medication!"

I turn back to Janni and Susan. I have no idea what to do.

"It's late. The office will be closed," I say stupidly.

"She needs to go the the hospital."

"Which one? Alhambra?" I shoot back. "She's not going to the hospital. Kids do weird things. I picked my gums as a kid until they bled."

"It's not the same thing!" Susan cries. "She's trying to kill herself."

"Will you stop saying that?" I yell back.

"What do you want me to say?" Susan demands, holding Janni in her arms. From the other bedroom, I hear Bodhi start to cry.

"Just give her a bath and get her to bed. I'll leave a message for Howe."

I leave Janni's room and retrieve the phone, dialing Howe's number. The after-hours message comes on, telling me, "If this is a life-threatening emergency, hang up and dial 911. Otherwise, please leave a message and your call will be returned on the next business day."

The message beeps at me. I open my mouth, but nothing comes out. What do I say? *Ah, yes, hi. This is Michael Schofield. My daughter is January Schofield. She wants to break her own neck. Can Doctor Howe please call me back at her earliest convenience?*

I hang up the phone

"Dial 911," the message said.

We already tried that once and that didn't help, either.

I don't know what to do anymore.

CHAPTER TWENTY-TWO

October 2008

I decide that Janni's attempt to strangle herself isn't serious, but just a way to avoid being put in time-out. All she needs to do is act like she is going to hurt herself and Susan will let her out, defeating the whole purpose of time-outs, which is to get Janni to think about why she got them in the first place. I am trying to connect consequence to action.

So I up the ante. When I come home from work, I usually have to make two dinners: one for me and Susan and another for Janni, because Janni won't eat what we eat. She will eat only mac 'n' cheese or cheese pizza.

That has to change.

Tonight, I make only one dinner for all of us, a rice dish, which I serve to Janni.

She looks down at it like it is a plate of worms. "I won't eat this."

"Well, that's dinner, Janni."

"I want mac 'n' cheese."

"You eat too much mac 'n' cheese."

"That's all I'll eat."

"You'll eat what I put in front of you," I answer, the words sounding unnatural coming out of my mouth.

Janni turns to Susan. "Mommy, make me mac 'n' cheese."

Susan starts to get up.

"No," I tell her forcefully. "No mac 'n' cheese. She has to eat what we're having."

Susan ignores me, pulling a box of microwave mac 'n' cheese from the freezer. "It's not that big of a deal."

"Yes, it is! She's got to learn to knuckle under."

"I was a picky eater when I was a kid. So were you. I remember your dad telling me that you wanted your food mashed up in a blender before you would eat it."

"That was just another part of my mother's craziness."

Susan puts the box in the microwave. "Maybe it wasn't. Maybe it was just you."

This makes me see red. "That's not the point. The point is you are letting her divide us. We need to be a united front. She needs to eat what we put in front of her. We're the adults, not her. If she doesn't eat, she doesn't eat. Eventually, when she gets hungry enough, she'll eat."

"I won't eat," Janni chimes in.

"Then you get nothing," I say to her.

"You're acting like your mother. I'm not going to starve her," Susan replies.

I turn away to avoid saying an expletive in anger. "Janni, sit at the table," I command.

"I'm not eating the rice."

"If you want the mac 'n' cheese, you need to eat some of the rice."

Janni picks up her spoon and shovels in a mouthful, then immediately leans over and spits it onto the floor.

"That's it," I say. "Time-out. Go to your room."

"I'm hungry!"

"Go!"

Janni picks up the plate of rice and dumps it on the floor. I grab her arm. "Let's go," I say. Janni lets her body go limp. Damn, she is too smart for her own good. She knows that going limp makes it harder for me to get her into her room because I have to pull her entire body weight. I won't pull on her arm for fear of dislocating it, so I pick up her legs and drag her across the carpet.

"You're not Ghandi," I tell her. I've taught her about Ghandi and nonviolent resistance. "This is not nonviolent resistance against oppression." I'm talking to her like an adult again, but it's only because of the "disconnect" between her mind and her body. If I don't punish her for a tantrum, all people will see is her behavior.

I pull Janni into her room and let go. "Ten minutes. You need to think about why you are in a time-out."

As I am walking past, she reaches up and hits me hard in the shin. "Twenty minutes now." I walk out and lock her bedroom door.

Nothing crashes against the door. Not that there is much left in her room. The beautiful room I made for her before she came home from Alhambra has been largely destroyed.

I put my ear up against the door, straining to hear any sounds that might tell me she is trying to choke herself.

Nothing. Once she tells me what she did, acknowledges it and owns her behavior, I will let her out.

"Janni, why are you in a time-out?"

A long silence. I don't think she's going to answer. This is the problem. She has to make the connection between cause and effect. For someone so brilliant, she seems to be unable to do this.

"I hit Bodhi."

This catches me by surprise, because that's not what she did.

"Well, that is usually why you get time-outs, because you *try* to hit Bodhi, but that's not what you did this time."

"I hit Mommy."

I'm getting annoyed. "No, you didn't hit Mommy," I say. "Stop playing games, Janni. The sooner you face what you did, the sooner you can come out."

"I screamed," Janni answers through the door.

"Well, yes, but that's not the main reason. Janni, what did you just do a second ago that got you a time-out? Just tell me and I'll let you out."

"I hit," Janni says again.

"Who? Who did you hit?"

"Bodhi."

"No."

"Mommy."

"No, Janni!" I reply, frustrated. "Janni, you could end all this right now. Just take responsibility for your actions."

"Tell me."

"No, I'm not going to tell you. If I tell you, that defeats the whole point of the time-out."

"Tell me. I don't remember."

"How could you not remember? You just did it a minute ago. It was the last thing you did."

"Let her out," Susan commands.

"No," I tell her, feeling like I am losing a battle. "She has to face the consequences."

"I don't remember," Janni says again through the door. "Just tell me what I did."

I open the door. Janni is sitting on her bed. I stare at her. "You deliberately spilled the rice and then hit me."

"Oh," Janni answers. "Can I come out now?"

I shake my head and walk away.

. . .

IT'S A SATURDAY in the middle of October and we're in sweltering heat running Honey around at Janni's school. Janni didn't want to come, but I told her she had no choice in the matter. There is no way I am leaving her alone with Susan and Bodhi.

A group of kids on bikes suddenly ride into the schoolyard, and I see Honey approaching them, picking up speed. This is not good. Honey doesn't bite, but she is a herding dog by instinct. If these kids aren't used to dogs and see one running toward them, they will get scared.

"It's okay," I call across the playground to them as Honey comes running. "She doesn't bite."

"Watch out for Wednesday," Janni suddenly calls. "She bites."

The kids turn to Honey, apprehension on their faces, and I realize they think Honey is Wednesday, Janni's imaginary rat.

"Janni, I wish you hadn't done that. Now they think Honey is Wednesday and they will be afraid."

"But I had to warn them about Wednesday," Janni protests.

"Janni, Wednesday can't hurt them," I answer, annoyed. "Honey! Get over here!"

"Yes, she can. She bites. She bites me."

"Dammit, Janni. I can assure you Wednesday cannot hurt them."

"Yes, she can. She can hurt them in their head."

This catches me so much by surprise that I forget about Honey scaring the other kids. I turn to Janni. She is looking at me like she finally has my attention.

"She bites me in my head if I don't do what she wants. That's why I have to hit Bodhi. If I don't, she will bite me."

She says this with total seriousness. That's it. Her imagination has gotten out of control. It controls her now.

"Janni, you control Wednesday, not the other way around. If she wants you to hit Bodhi, you tell her no."

"I do, but she won't listen and then she scratches me and bites me until I do."

This is ridiculous. "Janni, you created Wednesday! She's part of your imagination. You can tell her what to do!"

"No, I can't."

I feel myself losing control. "Janni, Wednesday doesn't exist, okay? She's a figment of your imagination. You can make her go away. Just tell her to go away!"

Janni shakes her head. "I can't."

"No. You won't. You won't because . . . because I don't know why." I pause, trying to decide how to proceed. I've been talking to her like she was an adult since she was a toddler. I know she has the capacity to understand what I am trying to say. "Because you can control Wednesday and make her do what you want, when playing with real kids requires give-and-take. You prefer your imaginary friends over real kids because you can control them and you can't control real kids. You can't control the real world, and that scares you. I get that, Janni. The real world is scary. But you're six years old now. It's time to give up your imaginary friends."

"They're not imaginary. They're real."

"I don't want to hear it, do you understand?" I wave my finger in her face. "I've had it with Calilini and all these friends of yours. I don't want to hear another word about them. I only want to hear about real people and real places." I am breathing hard. For three years I have played along. Not anymore. She's got to face reality now.

Janni stares at me, her face blank.

"They are real," she replies evenly, and walks away toward our car.

"Janni, come back here!"

She ignores me.

Whispers of guilt drift through me. This is my fault. I was so afraid of shutting down her imagination for fear of limiting her genius. I turned her into what she is, and now she probably feels I am rejecting her.

Susan told me that the other night, Janni said to her, "I wish I was dumb."

I start to run after her. "Janni, wait!" I have to call her several times before she turns around. "Make sure you have Wednesday."

Janni stares blankly for a second, then, "I do. See?" She raises her empty palm. "Squeak!"

"I see." She doesn't smile, but I see it in her eye, a fleeting look of happiness.

CHAPTER TWENTY-THREE

November 2008

I cancel my classes today so I can attend Janni's "IEP," or "Individualized Education Plan," meeting with Susan at Janni's school. The primary purpose of an IEP is to determine whether a child meets the requirements for special education services. Originally, when we requested it a month ago, our goal was to get them to provide Janni with a more challenging curriculum, with the hope that something would spark her interest and she'd want to study it on her own.

We are in a conference room with the principal, Mrs. Fitzgerald, the assistant principal, Wendy, Oak Hills' school psychologist, and Janni's first-grade teacher, Mrs. Parris. Usually, IEPs are done after class hours, but since we have no one to watch Janni, we asked if it could be done while Janni was in class and a substitute was filling in.

I can't help but notice they're all on one side of the table. Susan and I take up the empty seats opposing them, with Bodhi in between us sleeping in his stroller. I don't know if this arrangement happened purely by accident, but it adds to the feeling that this is going to be us against them.

"Janni is telling us she isn't getting to go to recess," Susan tells them accusingly.

I give an exasperated sigh. Susan does this every time we meet with the school. She is always immediately combative.

"Let's give Mrs. Parris a chance to speak," I say.

"She does get bench time occasionally," Mrs. Parris answers flatly.

"What is 'bench time'?" I ask.

"If a student breaks a rule, they get one warning. If they do it again, they lose their recess privileges and have to stay in and think about what they did."

I get an image of Janni, sitting on the bench, watching the other kids play.

"And does it work?" I ask rhetorically, because I know it doesn't. I've been doing it at home for six months, and it hasn't worked for me.

"No, it doesn't," she sighs, then turns to Susan. "Mrs. Schofield, can I ask you a question?" Without waiting for an answer, she continues. "Every time I take away a privilege—"

"Recess is not a privilege for Janni," Susan says, interrupting. "I don't know if you realize this, but Janni can't stop moving, and to take away recess from her is just torture. It's not like she even plays with the kids."

"Putting that aside for a moment," Mrs. Parris continues. "Janni says 'It's okay. My mommy will take me to Pizza Kitchen.' Is that true?"

"Yes, it is," Susan replies. "I do it because it is the only place she will eat. I'm not going to starve her."

Mrs. Parris exhales. "It just makes it harder for me to discipline Janni if she knows that no matter what I do, she is going to get the reward of going to Pizza Kitchen."

"Well, can you get her to eat the lunch I pack for her here?" Susan fires back.

"No," she admits.

"She can't control it!" Susan yells, looking at each of the school personnel in turn. "She has a mental illness!"

I sigh. "We don't know that."

Susan glares at me like I'm stupid. "She's tried to choke herself."

"That's because she knows it will get her out of a time-out."

Susan snorts and turns away from me, disgusted. "You can believe what you want. If you want to be stupid like them, fine."

I grit my teeth. Now she is calling me names, which doesn't help. "We are trying to find a solution here."

"We know what the solution is, but they won't do it," Susan retorts. "Janni needs more challenging work! She's a genius, but these idiots don't seem to get that."

I turn away, fighting to stay calm. Susan looks like a nut right now.

"Mrs. Schofield, we want to help," the principal says, "but insulting my staff is not helping. I can assure you," he continues, "that Mrs. Parris is an excellent teacher. I handpicked all my teachers. They are the best."

Bodhi stirs in his car seat, and Susan picks him up and cradles him in her arms, probably because he's the only one who is comforting to her in this moment.

"Look," I say, putting my hand on Susan's before she calls the principal an idiot, as well, "I am sure she is an excellent teacher under normal circumstances." I'm lying, and not very convincingly. The job of a teacher is to inspire, and there is nothing inspirational about Parris. "Janni is very sensitive. If she *perceives* that Mrs. Parris doesn't like her, the relationship is over."

"It's not a perception," Susan says, getting in her dig.

"That's not true," Mrs. Parris answers evenly. "I like January very much. When I am working one-on-one with her, she's a wonderful student. But I have sixteen other students who need my help. It's frustrating for me, because while Janni does understand the material, most of my other students do not. They need my help more than Janni. But as soon as I leave to go on to another student, Janni refuses to do her work, work I know she can do. Worse than that, she becomes disruptive, screaming and throwing things."

"She has a 146 IQ," Susan jumps in, her body jerking so much she wakes up Bodhi, who's been sleeping in her arms.

"We know how bright she is," the principal says. "As part of the IEP process we did a battery of tests. We weren't able to get as much information as we would have liked because of Janni's limited cooperation, but we learned enough to know she is the smartest student in this school, maybe the district."

"There you go," Susan says triumphantly.

"But," the principal continues, "none of that matters if she can't function within the classroom setting."

Can't function. In my mind, I see the image of Janni's future as a shut-in, just as I did when she was at Violet's party a couple years ago.

"I didn't want to say this," Mrs. Parris goes on, "but I just completed parent-teacher conferences, and several parents complained about Janni. They're upset their children are coming home and saying they can't learn because she's always screaming or disrupting the class."

Cold anger makes me shiver. *Other parents are complaining about my child?* Instinctively, my parental desire to protect my child kicks in. "And what did you tell them?" I ask coldly.

Mrs. Parris shrugs. "I told them I do my best to make sure every student gets the attention he or she needs, but I have to be honest. They don't. Janni takes up more of my time than is fair to the rest of the class. Even the other children are starting to avoid her."

"That's because they are picking up on your lead," Susan fires across the table.

Mrs. Parris shakes her head. "I go out of my way to make sure the other students include Janni. But it's hard for them, because she is extremely unpredictable. They want to play with her. They like her, but honestly I think they've given up trying to include her."

I look away. Emotions are surging to the surface; all my doubts, fears, and frustrations are overwhelming me.

"What about skipping her ahead to a higher grade?" I finally ask.

"I don't think that would be a very good idea," the principal answers.

"My biggest issue is getting her to write," Parris adds. "She knows how to do it, but she won't. The amount of writing only increases in the higher grades."

"And then there is the socialization issue," the principal continues. "We are not sure she would integrate well into an older classroom."

"But she needs kids more on her level," Susan says.

"She may be on their level intellectually, but not emotionally," the principal replies. "She's been in my office many times and I've gotten to know her. She spends most of her time talking about her imaginary friends. My fear is that putting her in with older kids would isolate her further than she already is.

"Look," the principal continues, "we all want the same thing, for Janni to succeed and be happy in her environment. I know you feel she would do better in a higher grade or even with another teacher, but given Janni's behavior issues and classroom disruptions, I don't see any evidence to support that."

"So you're going to do nothing," Susan says derisively, "while she gets worse and worse. Maybe when she runs out of the classroom and into the parking lot and gets hit by a car, then you'll do something."

"Susan," I say. "That's not helping."

She turns on me. "She's already tried to run before. They just happened to catch her in the parking lot. But what happens when they eventually aren't able to catch her? You keep thinking they care. They don't. If she dies, they'll just say, 'Oh, how awful! If only there was something we could have done.' We'll be the ones with a dead daughter!"

"I wish you wouldn't talk like that," I answer, as evenly as I can. "You make it sound like it's inevitable."

"It is! I can see it happening!"

The principal holds up his hand. "Our answer is not to do nothing. We agree Janni needs more than a mainstream classroom can provide . . ."

As soon as I hear *mainstream classroom,* I know where this is going.

The principal leans forward. "We feel the best placement for Janni at this time would be in an SED classroom."

"What's 'SED'?" I ask. Everything in public education is a damn acronym.

"Severely emotionally disturbed," the principal replies.

The conference room goes deadly quiet. I remember what my therapist Tom said last year . . . *It sounds like she is pretty disturbed.*

I shake my head vehemently. "No. No way. I know those classrooms. You're going to put her in with the kids who smoke and swear at the teacher. No way. That will send her backward, not forward. She needs someone to teach to her level." Anger and pain, emotions I haven't allowed myself to feel in months, are boiling up inside me. They don't want to help her. They don't value her. They just want her out of their hair. "You want to get rid of her because some other parents complained! Janni has a right to the same education as them!" I feel like I'm fighting for Janni's future now. If Susan and I don't hold our ground, if Janni gets sent to this classroom, it will be the beginning of the end. "She needs someone to teach her!" I say, staring daggers at Mrs. Parris. I wish to hell I had the time to teach Janni. These morons don't see her potential. All they can see is her behavior.

The principal puts up his hand. "That's not true, Mr. Schofield. It's a class for students with emotional and behavioral issues that require more than what a traditional classroom can offer. She could get the one-to-one attention there that we can't provide."

"What about a one-to-one here?" I ask.

"We don't feel that would be sufficient."

"You haven't tried it!" I am practically shouting. "Try it. The law says you have to exhaust all available options to keep her in a mainstream class before you can send her to an SED classroom."

The principal and his team exhange looks. "That is true," he finally answers.

"So you have to try a one-to-one and you haven't. That's what we want in Mrs. Parris's class."

"She isn't happy in a regular classroom," the principal replies. "Why make her suffer?"

I shake my head. *No. You just want to get rid of her.* "Do what Susan and I have to do every day. Keep trying. Get her a one-to-one."

The principal looks at Mrs. Parris, then back to us. "Okay."

I stand up. I'm not going to let them throw away Janni's potential because she's "difficult." Einstein was "difficult," too.

CHAPTER TWENTY-FOUR

December 2008

It's Winter Break and Janni is done with school for three weeks, which means a vacation from having to deal with Mrs. Parris and the endless calls from the school about Janni's behavior.

Once again I have brought Honey up to the school grounds to run and made Janni come with me. It's after dark and the school grounds are empty. The playing field is fenced in, so I can let Honey off her leash to run.

"Honey!" I hold up a tennis ball. I need Honey to burn off some energy to tire her out.

Honey comes over, but I don't throw the ball. I want to get her worked up enough for the ball so she'll go chasing it.

"Come on, Honey! Jump!" I hold the ball out and she goes for it. But then I pull it up higher, out of her reach, forcing her to jump for it. I do this repeatedly until Honey is absolutely berserk, and then I heave it into the darkness and Honey runs after it.

Janni is swinging by herself. She says she rarely gets to swing at school because there's a twenty-second time limit. I hate watching her swing by herself.

Janni gets off the swings and crosses to the tetherball and four-square courts.

I look over at Honey, who can't find the ball. She trots off toward Janni.

I start across the field, hoping I can find the ball in the dark.

"Ow!" I hear Janni cry out.

"What happened?" I ask, turning and running toward her, nervous. Did she trip?

"Honey stepped on my foot."

I slow, relaxing. "Oh." That's no big deal. Honey only weighs about forty-five pounds and is already trotting off after another scent.

But then I see Janni walking briskly after her, her arm up in the air.

"Janni," I call. "What are you doing?"

"I have to hit her." She says this like it's a fact.

"Janni, it was an accident. Honey didn't mean it."

"Yes, she did."

"How could she have meant it? She's a dog."

Honey is still trotting along, sniffing, oblivious to Janni, who's coming up behind her, fist in the air.

"Janni!" I yell from a hundred feet away. "Do not hit Honey!"

"I have to," she answers, as if she's in pain and this is the only way to relieve it.

"Honey!" I scream to her. "Run!" I race toward Honey. I don't know how hard Janni will hit Honey, if it will be only a light slap or if she'll hit Honey repeatedly. Not that it matters. I can't allow her to get away with hurting an animal. There was a time when Janni would never hurt an animal, but I don't have time to think about that now.

Honey looks up and sees me coming full tilt. Thinking it's a game, she runs off, Janni's fist missing her by inches.

Janni turns to follow Honey, but I reach her, grabbing her arm.

"Let me go," she says flatly.

"Janni, it was an accident."

"I have to hit her."

"No, you don't."

"Yes, I do." Janni tries to pull free from me, while Honey's sniffing grass twenty feet away.

"Janni, I can't let you hit Honey."

Janni turns to me, as if just realizing that it's me holding her back, but she's not looking at my face, just down at my chest.

She hits my arm and then my chest, her fist raining down heavy blows on me. I am so used to this by now that the pain barely registers.

"I need to hit her," Janni tells me as if I just can't understand.

I stand between her and Honey. "Then you are going to have to get past me," I say playfully, like this is a game of tag rather than my daughter trying to hurt her beloved dog.

I present myself as an alternate target. Better me than Honey. The last thing I want is Honey starting to fear or distrust Janni. I couldn't deal with that. "Bet you can't get me," I say to taunt her.

Maybe she'll get angry enough with me that she'll be distracted from Honey. If I can get her to chase me instead of Honey, I can run until she gets tired. I challenge her, praying it will work. Janni swings her fist at me, but I jump back. "Come on," I taunt playfully. "Come get me."

She starts running after me. I feel relief. My plan is working. She comes within three feet of me, close enough that I can see her dull eyes. Not the eyes of my daughter, but I have no time to think about that right now, either. Her fist is flying toward me. I step back, out of range, and jog a few feet backward, still facing her.

"Come on, you can do better than that!"

Just as she reaches me, I jerk away. I feel her fist slice down my side. I laugh. "Hah, hah. Missed me!"

I scuttle a few feet, looking back over my shoulder to make sure she is chasing me and not Honey, who I can see crossing the field.

Janni spots her and immediately turns from chasing me to running toward Honey. She still hasn't forgotten. It's like Honey killed her family and she must exact revenge. I run toward Honey, my shoes pounding on the grass, and jump in between her and Janni.

"Janni. Hit me!"

"I have to hit Honey."

"I want you to hit me." I draw in close to her. "Come on, hit me."

Janni swings at me and I dance away like a boxer. "Come on," I call. "It's a free hit. No time-out. But you have to catch me first."

I start running her in circles, thinking she'll eventually figure out that she can get me if she crosses the circle, but she never breaks from my path.

Something is wrong. She's not getting tired. And I am. I leave the circle and jog backward, pulling out my cell phone to check the time. Twenty minutes have passed. I turn and break into a dead run to create enough separation so I can stop for a second and take a breather.

I reach the end of the field and turn back, breathing hard. My leg muscles are screaming in pain. I can't do this much longer. I look up at Janni, still coming. *She's not stopping.*

Suddenly, she turns away from me and starts after Honey again. I break into a sprint, ignoring the pain in my legs and the growing cramp in my side, until I get between her and Honey.

"Hah!" I gasp. "Not gonna let you do it." She comes right at me, fist raised. But I am too tired to run anymore. I stand still as she hits my arm and then my stomach.

"Come on! You hit like a girl!"

But she is changing direction, running toward Honey again.

"Honey!" Janni calls. "Come here, Honey!" It sounds like *"Here's Johnny!"* from *The Shining.*

Honey turns, complying.

"No, Honey!" I labor after Janni.

"Honey, come here," Janni calls.

No. Now she is trying to lure Honey close enough to hit her. It is so evil, so out of character for her, but again I push it out of my mind.

I reach Janni and put my arms around her as we both fall back onto the ground, pulling her back on top of me.

She tries to break free.

"I need to hit Honey."

"No, you don't."

"Yes, I do."

The back of her head slams into my nose, on purpose or by accident I'm not sure. But in shock I let go and she's up on her feet again, going after Honey.

"Janni," I weakly call after her. "Come hit me. Hit me instead of Honey."

But Janni ignores me, and Honey is coming over to see what we're doing.

I stagger to my feet and give chase, catching Janni around the waist and bringing her down again. I wrap her in my arms. She kicks at my legs and hits me in the face with the back of her head.

"Just let me hit Honey!"

"I can't do that, Janni. She's an innocent dog."

"Just let me do it!"

She wriggles free, and I pull myself to my knees and grab her, bringing her back down to the grass. I pin her arms.

She isn't going to stop. How the hell am I going to get them both home without Janni hitting Honey? I brought them here for a little fun, and now I'll have to call Susan to come up here so Honey can ride in her car, and I'll take Janni. But she has Bodhi. I don't want to drag Bodhi out in this cold night air.

I get to my feet and lift Janni off the ground, so I am not dragging her over concrete, and start the long walk back to the car in the parking lot, with her continually beating me about the head. I'm emotionless, with just a single thought: *Get her to the car.*

We reach the car and I put her in the backseat. It will be easier for me to protect Honey if she's the one in the front now. I can use my arm as a shield. Janni gets one final punch in, this time on my mouth. It hurts, but I just close the door.

I have no idea where Honey even is now. I can't see her in the dark, as I silently curse myself for coming up here.

"Honey!" I yell into the night a few times before she reappears.

I put her leash back on and open the front passenger door. Honey hops up and I close the door.

As I am moving around the front of the car, the dome light is on from the door just being opened, and I see Janni lean forward from the backseat. She lifts her fist and brings it down on Honey's nose before I can even make it into the driver's seat.

Honey flinches but otherwise doesn't react.

I wrench open the door, ready to leap between Janni and Honey. But Janni is done. She's now staring straight ahead, ready to go home, as if nothing happened.

She was right. She just needed to hit Honey.

I failed to stop Janni from hitting Honey. It was just one hit this time, but what about next time? What do I do? Leave Janni at home, exposing Bodhi to her, or bring her out with me and risk her hitting Honey?

I look up at the starless sky. I don't know anymore. I just want to get everybody home, Janni to bed, and end another day in this hell we're living in.

CHAPTER TWENTY-FIVE

Christmas Day, 2008

Our friend Dave and his eleven-year-old son, Cameron, are coming over to spend Christmas Day with us. Dave works at KFI Radio, which was my first job when I arrived in LA in the mid-nineties. Dave was there when Susan and I first met thirteen years ago, seemingly a lifetime ago. Susan recently reconnected with him through the Internet and started talking to him about our problems with Janni.

We hadn't seen him in years, but he could relate because his son, Cameron, also has "issues" and is on medication for Asperger's and bipolar disorder. I get the sense that Susan feels she can talk to Dave easier than she can talk to me. She's also been commiserating with her friend Tracy from her old workplace, since she has kids on the Autistic spectrum. All three of them talk on Facebook now. Susan still believes there is a mental illness involved, but I don't want to hear this. There is no point. Even if Janni does have a mental illness, there is no one to help her except us.

MICHAEL SCHOFIELD

Nonetheless, I like it when Dave and his son come over, because when Janni loses it, he doesn't bat an eye. There's no judgment or shock. He knows what it's like to be attacked by your own child.

We're going out for dinner, but first I have to take Honey out, and with Dave here I can actually take her for a real walk, a full walk, not the usual racing Honey through her business. Dave will be here to help if Janni goes after Bodhi. He is the only person on earth I trust to leave Janni alone with Susan and Bodhi.

Except that this time Janni wants to come, and so does Cameron, meaning Dave will come, too. I should say no. Honey is great with other dogs, but not so great with humans other than us.

But I agree, too tired to deal with Janni's meltdown and violence if I say no.

I walk a few feet ahead of the others so Honey keeps her focus on sniffing the ground and disregards Dave and Cameron.

We've only gone a hundred yards when Janni suddenly stops.

"I can't go on." She drops down onto the asphalt of the parking lot and lies there.

Shit. I can't carry her back and hold Honey at the same time, and I can't hand Honey to Dave because she will lunge at him, even if she doesn't bite. She is a nipper.

"Come on, Janni. Just a little farther."

"No."

"Janni, you said you wanted to come. We have to keep going. Honey needs to do her business."

"No."

I've been through this before. The best thing to do is to wait and act like this isn't annoying me in the least. Janni can never stay in one place for very long. Eventually, she'll get bored and decide to get up and keep going.

"I'll wait."

188

"I'm not going."

"That's fine."

"Never."

"Okay."

I wait, while still keeping my eyes out for cars that might come speeding through the parking lot.

Instinctively, as if reading my mind, Dave moves to where the parking lot curves, positioning himself as a human barrier. If a car races in, he'll be hit first.

"Janni, let's at least get out of the parking lot. You know cars can come through here pretty quick."

"No."

"I just don't want you to get run over."

Janni doesn't move. This is taking longer than usual. Maybe it's because I'm hungry, or maybe for just once I want to have a peaceful night, but I start to lose my patience.

"Janni, if you don't get up, we aren't going to Red Lobster."

Janni sits up and climbs to her feet. I relax, thinking I've enticed her. But she moves toward Honey, eyes down, dull. Her fist goes up in the air.

No, not again. Honey is on the leash, trapped. I turn my body to Janni, attempting to block her, but I get twisted up in the leash, pulling Honey closer. Janni hits Honey hard enough that I can hear the thud.

"Janni!" I retreat across the parking lot, trying to get Honey away, but Janni is still coming. She hits Honey again. Honey just puts her head down like she did something wrong. You would never know this was the same dog I had to hold off the sheriff's deputies last spring. Maybe, on some level, Honey knows this really isn't Janni.

Janni is still hitting Honey, and I can't protect her as long as she remains on the leash. I wish I could let her go, but Honey would just go after Dave and Cameron.

Dave steps toward us, ready to help, but Honey leaps to the end of her leash, barking and snarling at Dave, oblivious to Janni's hitting her.

"Janni," Dave calls softly. "Come over here with me and Cameron."

"Janni, don't do that," Cameron adds, watching her hit Honey. This bothers me even more. If he's disturbed by what Janni is doing to Honey, then Janni is worse than he is.

But Janni keeps on hitting Honey. I keep moving to face her, trying to put my body between Janni and Honey, but Honey, still on the leash, has nowhere to go except around me in circles. Janni keeps following her, like a carousel from hell.

"Do you want me to get her?" Dave asks.

I wish I could hand Honey off to him, but there is no way. Maybe Janni won't be violent with Dave.

"Okay, pick her up."

Dave grabs Janni, and she immediately hits him on the head.

"Janni, stop!" I order her.

"It's okay," Dave replies calmly. "I'm used to it. This is nothing."

I follow Dave back to our apartment, Janni hitting him and kicking him the entire way, Cameron walking next to his father, trying to coax her.

"Janni, calm down," he says. "You want to go to Red Lobster. You want to get mac 'n' cheese." One mentally ill child consoling another, while Honey is still barking and lunging at them, forcing me to pull her back on her leash.

We get back upstairs to our apartment.

"What happened?" Susan asks, watching Dave go past with Janni beating his head.

"She started hitting Honey for no reason." It's hard to talk over Honey's incessant barking at Dave and Cameron, whom she perceives as intruders.

"Where do you want her?" Dave asks. Janni is still whaling away at his head, knocking off his glasses.

"Susan, put Bodhi down so you can take Honey," I direct.

I take Janni from Dave and immediately the blows come down on my head. I walk into her room and put her down.

"Okay, time-out. You have to stay here until you calm down."

"I'm hungry!" she screams at me.

"We can't go until you calm down." I start to close the door, but Janni bolts for it. I stick out my hand and push her aside so I can lock the door. I know the time-outs don't change her behavior, but I just need a place to stash her so I can take Honey out.

Immediately something smashes into the door, probably her chair again.

"What now?" Dave asks.

"Did you take Honey out?" Susan asks.

"I never got the chance. She wouldn't go any farther than the parking lot. Honey still has to go."

"I'll take her out," Susan offers.

Another crash comes from behind Janni's door. I can't listen to this.

"No, I'll take Honey."

I SLOWLY WALK Honey around the complex, not wanting to go back, even though Janni has probably calmed down by now. But I know it's getting late, so I put Honey in the garage and head upstairs.

The first thing I see when I enter the apartment is Cameron at Janni's open bedroom door. He turns to me, tears streaming down his face.

"She stopped throwing things, so I asked if I could go in, and Susan said yes, and I went in, and Janni was falling out of the window . . ."

I race past him into Janni's bedroom. Susan is standing inside, holding Bodhi, crying. "Janni, please come back inside!" she begs.

Time slows down as I follow Susan's gaze to Janni's bedroom window.

It is open.

Dave's body is pressed up against the part of the sliding window that doesn't open, face red and perspiring, glasses retrieved but dangling from his face. He is straining to hold on to Janni's feet, wedged between his body and his left arm.

"I need to get away," I hear Janni screaming into the night through the open window. "Let me go! Let me go!"

My brain paralyzes. *Janni . . . is . . . trying . . . to . . . jump . . . out . . . the . . . window.* My daughter, my little girl, whom I used to shadow when she was a baby, protecting her from other kids, is trying to jump out the window, yet I can't react. I don't know how to react anymore.

"Janni!" I say weakly as Dave pulls her back through the window. His face red, he slams the window closed before sagging down the wall, spent.

"Janni, what were you doing?" I ask. Janni is trying to open the window. Dave struggles to his feet and holds it closed.

"I want to get away."

"Janni, you could have fallen on your head and died." My voice is so weak, like I am fading.

"I have to get away."

"From what?"

Janni suddenly turns from the window. "I'm hungry. Can we go to Red Lobster?"

I know I should press her to find out what the hell she was doing, but I don't. I'm afraid. I am afraid because she was trying to "get away." And whatever she was trying to get away from in here, alone in her room, is worse than dropping from a second-floor window.

CHAPTER TWENTY-SIX

December 29, 2008

I am sitting on the couch in Dr. Howe's office as Susan is describing how Janni tried to jump out the window.

I am thinking, but not about that. I can't bring myself to think about that. If I do, I know I will fall apart. I am supposed to be Janni's protector. I would give my life for her. Yet, when it happened, I was too numb to respond. But that numbness is the only thing that allows me to function.

Instead, I find myself thinking about when I was a kid. My dad had his private pilot's license, and he used to take me flying with him. He always made me feel like I was a real copilot by involving me in the process, and one of the most important jobs of the copilot is to read the various checklists to the PIC (pilot in command). It's a way of making sure the pilot has done everything he or she is supposed to do.

I remember reading the checklist to him. Everything I read, he would repeat, double-checking that the procedure had been done.

Fuel set to center?
Fuel set to center.
Mixture rich?
Mixture rich.
Engine cowls open?
Engine cowls open.
Master switch on?
Master switch on.

I think about my questioning of Janni, trying to get her to see the connection between her actions and the consequences.

What did you do?
I hit Bodhi.
No. What did you do?
I screamed.
No.

It's like she's guessing at the answer. . . .

Oh, my God.

"She's guessing," I suddenly say out loud.

"What?" Dr. Howe and Susan say simultaneously.

I stare at the floor. "Every time I put her in for a time-out, I tell her she can't come out until she takes responsibility and admits what she did that got her there in the first place, but she guesses at the answer and never gets it right. She always starts with 'I hit Bodhi,' then she'll say, 'I screamed,' and she keeps running down a checklist of everything she might have done until she gets the right answer."

I rub my eyes. "I always assumed she was playing a game, but now I realize she really doesn't know." I look Dr. Howe straight in the eye. "She's not playing. She really doesn't remember."

Dr. Howe appears lost in thought for a moment. She glances up at us, and I get the sense she is struggling with whether to tell us something.

"She doesn't remember," she finally says, "because she's dis-associating."

Disassociating. Doctor-speak. Part of their unique "language." I remember first learning this term in college psychology. Like most psychiatric terms, it doesn't sound particularly threatening. That's because Dr. Howe left off the rest of the sentence: *from reality.*

A person "disassociating" is a person who slides back and forth between two realities: ours and theirs.

"What does that mean?" Susan asks. I can hear the fear in her voice.

Dr. Howe looks over at Janni. "I think I might have been wrong about the mood disorder," she finally says. "I used to believe her psychosis was a product of her mood." She looks back at us. "Now I am starting to think it is the other way around. Her mood is the product of her psychosis."

"I don't get it," Susan says, darting her eyes between Dr. Howe and me.

"It's too soon to tell," Dr. Howe answers. "I really wish we could get her into UCLA, where they could observe her over a long period of time." *Observe her for what exactly?* She doesn't explain.

"What are you saying?" Susan knows something bad has been realized, just not what. I look over at Janni, at my little girl.

"Could be any number of things," Dr. Howe answers. "That's why she needs to be in UCLA."

Susan looks to me. She knows I know.

I sigh. "The first is bipolar with psychotic features. The second is schizophrenia."

Susan stares at me for a moment. I look down, unable to meet her eyes.

"So she does have schizophrenia," Susan says quietly, as if it is fact.

Dr. Howe, writing a prescription, shakes her head. "I didn't say that."

"Then what else could it be?"

Dr. Howe turns to us. "Remember what I told you when you first came in a year ago: The diagnosis is less important than the symptoms."

She tears a prescription off her pad and hands it to me. "I would like to try a low dose of Haldol."

Haldol. I know about Haldol. I've read about Haldol. In the movies where you see patients sitting in the corner, drooling, staring into space? That's Haldol.

"Haldol is used to treat schizophrenia," I say.

"It's a general treatment for psychosis," Dr. Howe answers, refusing to look at me.

"I've read about it. It's used only in the most extreme cases of schizophrenia where the patient has failed to respond to all other medications."

Susan turns to Dr. Howe, alarmed. "You mentioned Geodon before," she says, almost babbling with fear. "We haven't tried that yet."

Dr. Howe's face is impassive. "I don't think it would work. Risperdal had no effect on Janni, and Geodon is chemically very similar to Risperdal."

"It is schizophrenia, isn't it?" Susan says, her eyes tearing up. "I knew it."

"We can't say that yet," Dr. Howe replies.

But the dam has cracked. Dr. Howe can stick her finger in the crack all she wants, but there is no stopping the flood.

"Why not?" I ask. "What else is left?" Why can't Dr. Howe just admit it? Why maintain this sense of false hope? Schizophrenia has always been the potential eight-hundred-pound gorilla in the room, the worst-case scenario, but if she has it, just tell us. At least then we'll know. I look over at Janni, playing with the dollhouse. Let us enjoy what we have left of her.

"You can't just diagnose someone with schizophrenia," Dr. Howe responds.

"Why not?" I ask again.

"Because you just can't!" Dr. Howe snaps. I am taken aback, having never known her to be this flustered. "It takes a long period of observation to make that diagnosis, longer than a year."

She regains her composure, resuming writing on the prescription pad. "You might want to call your pharmacy and make sure they carry Haldol. It's not a commonly used antipsychotic anymore."

"Have you ever prescribed it before?" Susan asks.

Dr. Howe stops writing on her pad.

"Not to a child this young," she admits.

"Why?" I ask, even though I already can guess the answer.

Dr. Howe turns to me. "I've never had to."

Dr. Howe starts walking us out. Susan is in front, pushing Bodhi's stroller. Janni is next, followed by me, with Dr. Howe bringing up the rear.

"Give me a call in three days and let me know how the Haldol is doing," she says.

I nod.

She draws closer to me and whispers. "And keep seeing what you can do to get her into UCLA."

I stare at her and nod, still trying to process this.

CHAPTER TWENTY-SEVEN

January 12, 2009

I look across at Janni. It's her first day back at school. She is very quiet this morning. No mention of 400 or any of the others from Calalini.

I turn into the lot. "We're only five minutes late. If we hurry, you can get to class before Mrs. Parris does the absent list." I pull up in front of the school and pop my seat belt off.

"I can go by myself," Janni suddenly says, getting out of the car.

"Are you sure?" I ask, getting out and retrieving her roller bag from the backseat. I feel like I should go in with her, if for no other reason than to remind Mrs. Parris that I'm still here watching how she treats Janni.

"I'll be fine." Janni takes her backpack. She doesn't look upset; in fact, she just looks like any other child her age going to school. It occurs to me that I've never actually seen this.

"Wait a minute," I call to her.

She stops. I run up to her and give her a kiss on the top of the head. "I love you."

She kisses me back. "Love you." She turns and walks away, pulling her backpack behind her.

I get back in the car and call Susan.

"How was Janni when you dropped her off?" she asks.

"Fine. She didn't even complain about going to school this morning."

"Maybe the Haldol is working," she says with cautious optimism.

"It's too early to tell," I reply, unwilling to let myself feel any hope. "But she's never gone this long without talking about her imaginary friends."

I shift uncomfortably in my seat. "If the Haldol has taken away her imaginary friends . . ."

"Then that means they were never imaginary," Susan finishes my sentence.

When Janni told us at Loma Linda that the rats were afraid of Bodhi, she was telling the truth. They're real to her because they're hallucinations.

I AM WALKING into Walmart for cleaning supplies. My cell phone rings. I check the caller ID and it's the school district's main line.

I sigh. I just dropped her off twenty minutes ago.

"Hello, Mr. Schofield? It's Nancey from Oak Hills School. Janni was just brought into the nurse's office."

Janni must have gotten bored and requested to go to the nurse's office. I'm going to have to let Nancey in on the secret.

"I'm not worried. That's what we told her to do if she was having a hard time in class. She'll sit there a few minutes, get bored, and go back to class."

"Well, I'm little worried, Mr. Schofield. She seems pretty sick. She's also drooling."

"That's the medication," I reply, growing annoyed. I know what they want. They want me to come and take her off their hands. "The medication she's on increases saliva production," I add. "No big deal."

"She says she can't walk."

I'm getting angry. I don't believe Janni can't walk. She's a smart girl. She knows what to say to get into the nurse's office, just like she knew what to do to get back into Alhambra.

"The medication makes her tired. She'll be fine. Call me if she gets worse."

I hang up. If I stay on the phone, we will just go in circles, with Nancey continually trying to convince me to come get Janni. I need this time to get cleaning supplies. I can't shop with Janni.

I'm inside Walmart, trying to remember everything I need to get, when my cell phone rings again. This time it's Susan.

"Doe?"

"The school called me!" she says, panicked, and I can hear the windblast coming from her driving the car.

"Yeah, I know," I reply. "They called me, too."

"She's having a stroke!"

"What?"

"They said she is drooling and can't walk!"

I roll my eyes, surprised Susan would buy into this. "That's not a stroke. That's what they told me, too. They just want us to come take her off their hands."

"They called the paramedics!" Susan screams into the phone.

My annoyance at the school vanishes, replaced by fear.

"They're overreacting," I say, trying to convince myself as much as Susan. "This is no big deal."

"She can't move her left side! They've called the paramedics to take her to the hospital!"

I shake my head. I can't believe it. I won't believe it.

"I need you to meet me at the school and take Bodhi! I'm going to the hospital with her. Where are you?"

"Walmart. I'll be there in five minutes."

The windblast is gone. Susan hung up.

This is an overreaction. Janni is fine. She has to be fine, I tell myself, leaving the half-full shopping cart behind in the aisle and running for the exit.

AS I COME down the hill toward the school, I see an ambulance in the driveway. Paramedics are coming out of the school, wheeling Janni on the gurney, one holding up an IV bag.

I floor the accelerator and take the curve fast enough that the right wheels leave the pavement. What keeps running through my mind is the fact that I didn't go to her immediately. I didn't take this seriously. I thought this was nothing.

I abandon the car in the middle of the parking lot, the engine still on, as I run toward Janni. She is being loaded into the back of the ambulance. I am close enough now to see that there is an oxygen mask on her face. Susan steps in behind her, holding Bodhi in her arms.

The principal moves to intercept me. "She's going to be fine, Mr. Schofield," he says, holding up his hands to reassure me.

I blow past him. Susan sees me coming. I can see anger in her eyes that I didn't react. One paramedic, the driver, gets out and is about to close the doors when I get there.

"What is happening?!" I ask, panicked.

Susan gets up and hands me Bodhi. "She wasn't able to breathe," she says, looking at me with pure hatred. "She would have died had they not called paramedics."

The paramedic holds up his hands. "She'll be fine. She's developed dystonia. Your wife said she's on Haldol, and that can cause dystonia.

We got her on a Benadryl drip. She'll be fine now, but we're still taking her to Henry Mayo."

JANNI IS ALREADY looking better by the time the ER doctor comes over to us.

"What happened?" I ask.

"She developed what we call a dystonic reaction." He's looking in Janni's eyes. "It's a common reaction to antipsychotics, especially Haldol." He lifts Janni's arms and checks their rigidity.

"Can it be fatal?" I ask. If he says yes, I deserve to die. I should have been there.

"No, not at all," he replies. "It's scary to watch, but it's not fatal. It's caused by spasms in the neck and facial area. The tongue protrudes from the mouth, which is what causes the drooling. It's easily treated with Benadryl, which relaxes the muscles. We'll keep her on the Benadryl drip for a couple of hours and observe her, but she should be fine." He looks into her pupils. "She is already looking better from when she first came in." He turns back to us. "Your wife said she was on Haldol?"

"Yes," I answer dumbly.

"What's her diagnosis?" he asks.

"Psychosis not otherwise specified."

He nods. "And her regular psychiatrist didn't prescribe Cogentin?"

"No."

He frowns. "I'm surprised, because Cogentin or at least regular Benadryl is pretty standard practice for anyone given Haldol because of its tendency to do exactly this."

"SHE WENT INTO dystonia!" I yell at Dr. Howe over the phone. I feel guilty as hell, but the fact that Howe didn't prescribe Cogentin gives me someone else to get angry at.

"I'm surprised," Dr. Howe replies calmly.

"The ER doc said she needs something called Cogentin! Why didn't you prescribe that? Did you not know about that?" I again don't trust Dr. Howe. This is over her head. She can't handle Janni. We have stuck it out with her for more than a year even though she clearly never had a clue. I should have found a new psychiatrist long ago. I didn't because I didn't want to have to try and explain all over again what we were going through. I was too tired.

"I know about Cogentin," Howe answers. "Normally it's given along with Haldol to prevent dystonic symptoms."

"Then why didn't you prescribe it?" I shout into my phone.

"Because I've given her powerful medications before in doses she shouldn't be able to handle and they haven't worked," she answers softly.

The anger in me dies like it was shot.

"Janni has the highest resistence to medication of anyone I have ever treated," Dr. Howe continues. "With any other patient I would have been worried about dystonia, but I didn't think it would be a problem for Janni. I was wrong."

I close my eyes, thinking back to the ">99.9%" on Janni's IQ scores. I always knew Janni was unique. This is not how I wanted her to be unique.

CHAPTER TWENTY-EIGHT

Friday, January 16, 2009

My cell phone rings. I look down at the Caller ID, expecting it to be Susan, updating me on Bodhi. She's at the pediatrician with Bodhi for his one-year vaccinations.

But it is the school district main line again.

This is the first call from the school since Janni went into dystonia earlier in the week. The Haldol was lowered on Tuesday. Mrs. Parris had told us that Monday, prior to going into dystonia, Janni was the best she'd ever seen her. Tuesday, Janni did pretty well at school. Wednesday, she did okay. Thursday was like she was never on the Haldol at all.

"Mr. Schofield, this is Mrs. Fitzgerald. We need you to come get Janni."

"If she is showing signs of dystonia, give her Benadryl," I reply. "You have the letter from Dr. Howe authorizing you to dispense it."

"It's not that. Janni's exhibiting behavior that is very alarming to us."

I don't ask what the behavior is. I'm sure it's what we see every day.

"We called your wife, but she is refusing to come get her."

I know why Susan's refusing to come get her, and it has nothing to do with Bodhi needing his vaccinations. It's the same reason I don't want to go. Nobody will help Janni. Even at the hospital on Monday, we couldn't get someone to talk to us about what options we had. The social worker there said there were, once again, no beds available at UCLA; we wanted her to go as an inpatient for observation on the Haldol. Even the doctor who treated her thought she should be an inpatient, but we were told there was nothing they could do to help.

"She's at the doctor with our son."

"I understand that," Mrs. Fitzgerald replies, "but one of you needs to come get Janni right now."

"Is she hurt?"

"No, but her behavior is out of control."

I grin sickly into the phone. *Welcome to our world.*

"It'll be out of control at home, too."

"Mr. Schofield, somebody needs to come get her immediately."

No, I think. *You are not getting off the hook that easy.* "Doesn't the law require you to take responsibility for her during school hours?"

"No, Mr. Schofield, not if her behavior is disruptive to the functioning of the school."

It figures that even the law is not on our side. But if I come get her, what do I do with her? Bring her home? Then what? It suddenly hits me that I can't go on living like this. It's killing all of us, Janni included. We have struggled for more than a year on our own. This has to end.

"What happens if I don't?"

"Then we'll have to call the sheriff's office and report her abandoned."

This shocks me. I wonder if she is bluffing. Is this some kind of sick threat to get me to come take Janni off their hands? "You'd really do that?"

"Yes, if I have to, but I'd much rather you come and get her."

I pull the phone away from my ear and rub my face. To my great shock, part of me wants Mrs. Fitzgerald to call the police. I run through what would happen. Janni would be turned over to the care of the state. She would become their problem, whether they liked it or not. Maybe then she would finally get the help she needs. But she would be without us. She is my daughter. While I don't think she can feel fear anymore, I can't let go of the slim possibility that if I let her be taken by the state, one day she might snap out of this and her mommy, daddy, and little brother won't be there.

"Mr. Schofield, are you still there?"

"Yeah, I'm here."

"Are you coming?"

"I'm coming."

I GET OUT of my car and see Mrs. Fitzgerald exiting the school to meet me. "I was worried you weren't coming."

"I said I was coming," I say, with no pretense of politeness.

"I wasn't sure from our phone conversation," she says as we enter the building.

I always come. I am her father.

"What happened?"

She opens the door to the main office. "She started running around the school, trying to throw herself through doors and windows."

Through doors and windows? I think skeptically. This woman is really trying to sell this thing. She probably just ran out of the classroom in such a rage that she couldn't control her motor skills enough to get the door open, like what happens when she's in time-out at home.

Mrs. Fitzgerald is still speaking. ". . . like they weren't even there. We were terrified she was going to hurt herself."

"Where is she now?" I ask as we enter the main office. But before she can answer, I see Janni through the window of Mrs. Fitzgerald's office, or what used to be her office.

"It took us a while, but we finally managed to herd her into my office. We removed everything she can throw, so she can't hurt herself. She's safe for now, but we need to talk about what we're going to do."

I peer in and see Janni standing next to the desk, gesturing to a woman I've never seen before, who is sitting in Mrs. Fitzgerald's chair, drawing a picture on a piece of paper. Another woman I don't know is leaning up against the rear door of the office. I look around the room. The office, usually filled with books and old toys, is now barren, just like the quiet room back at Alhambra.

Instinctively, I reach for the door handle, but it won't move.

Mrs. Fitzgerald comes over, keys in her hand. "The door is locked for her own protection."

This is no exaggeration. This is really happening. They are scared enough either for Janni or themselves to actually lock her in an office.

She unlocks the door and I rush in. "Janni, are you okay?"

The woman sitting next to Janni, drawing, looks up and smiles. "Hi, I'm Karen, one of the district psychologists."

"I've instructed two people to be with Janni at all times," Mrs. Fitzgerald tells me.

"We're drawing a picture of 400," Janni tells me, rubbing her hands together excitedly. I stare at her, trying to understand the happy girl I'm seeing inside this bare, guarded office.

"We're doing fine." Karen smiles up at me, showing none of the fear Mrs. Fitzgerald does. "She's telling me what 400 the Cat and Magical 61 look like, and I'm drawing them for her."

"Magical 61 is here," Janni says happily. "She came to meet me."

Jesus Christ, Janni. You are locked in an office. Don't you realize that? She is acting like this is completely normal.

"Do you want to see Magical 61?" Janni asks me. "She's a girl like me, except she's eight."

A girl like me. There is no one like you. That's the problem.

"She's right there." She points behind me, but I don't bother turning around.

"We should talk," Mrs. Fitzgerald whispers in my ear.

"I don't want to leave Janni."

"It's okay," Karen says, "Janni's teaching me about all her friends."

This surprises me. She didn't say "imaginary friends." Only "friends." I have never met anybody other than me who treats them as real.

"We can talk in the principal's office," Mrs. Fitzgerald tells me.

"Janni, I'll be in the next room if you need me, okay?"

"Okay." She turns her attention back to Karen's drawing.

I walk into the principal's office, dulled. Mrs. Fitzgerald follows me, as does Wendy, the Oak Hills School psychologist, closing the door behind us.

I stand, unsure what to do.

"You can sit down," Mrs. Fitzgerald tells me and sits down in the principal's chair.

"Well, she seems okay now," I say.

"We have every school psychologist in the district here," Mrs. Fitzgerald says.

"Well, maybe they can go back to class with her, help her through the rest of the day. That's what she needs. At home she's fine as long as I give her the one-on-one attention," I babble.

"She can't go back to class, Mr. Schofield."

Her tone shocks me like ice water down my back.

"I can't let her back in school like this."

I stare, blankly. They don't just want me to take her home. They want me to keep her there.

"When can she come back?" I ask.

"Whenever she is no longer a threat to herself or others."

I look down at my legs. I can't believe this is happening. I feel like I got switched into someone else's body by mistake.

"She can't come to school like this, when she's this unstable," Mrs. Fitzgerald continues.

"It took the entire staff to chase her down. Teachers had to leave their classrooms to help. We had to lock down the classrooms. We can't go on like this."

"Neither can we." I want to cry, but no tears will come.

"She's suspended from Oak Hills until she stabilizes or we can get her transferred to the SED classroom," Mrs. Fitzgerald says.

I put my head in my hands. "How long will that take?"

"We need to have another IEP," she replies.

This is my fault. I was so terrified of her being labeled and marginalized that I refused to allow a transfer. And now this has happened.

I look up. "What you just saw? That's what we live with every day. Just last month she tried to jump out of her bedroom window. It was only because my friend was there that she didn't succeed."

Mrs. Fitzgerald says nothing. I realize I'm begging her. For what, I don't know. *Help. Please, somebody help us.*

"If I take her, nothing will change," I say quietly. "We will go home and it will just be the same."

"So you are not going to take her?" Mrs. Fitzgerald asks, seemingly shocked. "You realize we'll have to call the police?"

I look down, unable to bear what I'm considering. "What will happen to her if I let the police take her?"

I can feel Mrs. Fitzgerald and Wendy looking at each other. They weren't expecting this.

"I don't know," Mrs. Fitzgerald answers. "I assume they'll turn her over to the care of the county. I don't know what happens after that."

I can't bring myself to look them in the eye. Maybe out of shame. In my wildest dreams, I never thought it would come to this. I thought I would always be there for her.

I even came here today intending to take her back home, but now that the moment is here, I can't do it. I can't just take her home and go on trying to live. *We are not functional.*

"Mr. Schofield, what do you want to do?"

Every instinct in my body tells me to get up and take Janni home. But if I do, nothing will change. I've tried to save Janni all her life and I can't. I'm not enough. She needs more.

"Call the cops," I say quietly.

I AM NUMB.

Through the open door of the principal's office, I hear an LA County sheriff's deputy talking to Mrs. Fitzgerald.

"She's six years old!" he says. "I didn't know she was only six! I can't put a six-year-old in the back of my car. It's designed for criminals! There isn't even padding back there!"

"The father doesn't want to take her home. He doesn't think he can safely take her in the car."

The deputy comes into the room. "Mr. Schofield, I'm Deputy Dorman. I understand you don't want to transport your daughter for safety reasons, but I can call an ambulance to take her."

I slowly lift my eyes from the 9mm Beretta strapped at his side up to his face. "If you call an ambulance, they'll just take her to the nearest hospital, which is Henry Mayo. Henry Mayo doesn't have a psych unit. I know. We were just there on Monday." My voice is flat, robotic.

He looks from Mrs. Fitzgerald to me, then back again, clearly exasperated. He doesn't know what to do. I understand. Neither do I anymore.

He sighs. "Okay. I'm gonna be honest with you. I have no idea what to do in this kind of situation. I've never dealt with anything like this."

I start to fear that he, too, will leave us to struggle on alone, just as everyone else has.

Dorman gets out his cell phone. "I tell you what. I'm going to make some calls. We'll figure something out." He puts the phone to his ear. "I'm not going to leave until this situation is resolved, okay?"

I fight the desire to get up and embrace him. He isn't leaving. He isn't passing the buck. Nine months ago, two LA County sheriff's deputies were all ready to arrest me for allegedly molesting Janni. Now this deputy is my only hope.

Janni comes bounding into the room, followed by Karen.

"She wanted to come see you," Karen tells me.

"That's fine." I reach out to Janni, trying to pretend like this isn't happening, like I am not actually looking for someone to take her. "Hey, sweetie."

Karen sits down next to me. "How are you doing?"

"Not well."

"I can imagine."

Janni laughs at an empty spot on the carpet of the office. "Magical 61 is so funny. She's dancing in the office. Magical 61, you can't dance here!"

Deputy Dorman breaks off from the phone for a moment. "Hey, Janni. Who is Magical 61?"

Janni turns to him, as if seeing him for the first time. "She's my friend."

"Where is she?"

Janni turns and points at an empty corner of the office. "She's right there."

"Is Magical 61 real?"

Janni's smile evaporates. "No."

"So she's not real."

"No."

Karen leans over to me. "Did you teach her to say that?" she whispers.

"Say what?" I'm barely able to comprehend anything anymore.

"Answer that way when somebody asks her if her friends are real?"

Despite myself, I laugh. "There is no controlling what Janni says."

"I just wondered if you had coached her to do that."

"No," I chuckle. "Why?"

Karen lowers her voice even further. "Because it sounds like a canned answer, like she is saying what she thinks she is supposed to say. What's her diagnosis?"

"Well, it was bipolar with psychotic features, but now it is psychosis NOS."

She leans in even closer. "That surprises me."

"Why?"

"Because I've worked with adults like her before, and Janni's behavior looks like classic schizophrenia to me."

I stare at her. It feels like the clouds just parted and God spoke. Even Dr. Howe refused to apply the word directly to Janni, as if by not using the word we could all pretend it didn't exist.

"Thanks, Bert," Deputy Dorman says into his phone. "I really appreciate this." He hangs up and comes over to us. "There's this county service, the Psychiatric Emergency Team. I've never worked with them before, but they come when we have noncriminal psychiatric cases. They have a main number, but if you call, all you get is a message. I had to call pretty much everybody I've ever worked with." He smiles. "But I got a cell number for one of the team members."

LOS ANGELES COUNTY is the most populated county in the United States, with more than nine million people, spread out over an area larger than the states of Delaware and Rhode Island combined. There are eight two-person psychiatric emergency teams, or "PET Teams," for the entire county, or one team for every 1.2 million people. I didn't even know they existed.

Thirty minutes later, a small Hispanic woman named Maria arrives, alongside a huge, hulking white guy named Paul, both wearing county badges on chains around their necks.

Maria goes into Mrs. Fitzgerald's office to talk to Janni while Paul waits with me.

Paul's right eye is swollen, filled with blood. The right side of his face is purple with the largest bruise I've ever seen.

"What happened to your eye?" I ask.

Paul looks down at me. "I walked into a door," he answers, never batting an eye.

I realize the purpose of the PET team is to take people to psychiatric care, even when they don't want to go.

"Looks like that door put up a fight."

His face remains impassive. "Sometimes they do."

Maria comes out.

"So what's the situation?" I ask her, worried. Judging by the look on Paul's face, they're used to raving lunatics. I'm not sure they'll take Janni's situation seriously.

"We're gonna take her," she replies.

I breathe a sigh of relief.

"Where we going?" Paul asks.

Maria looks up at me. "Normally we would take her to the closest acceptable facility."

"That's Alhambra," I say.

"Probably."

"No. I don't want her to go there. It's UCLA or nothing." I am dead set about this. Two hours ago I was ready to give her up to the county. But now maybe, just maybe, the sun is breaking through. "Every time we call UCLA, they always say there are no beds available."

Maria smiles. "UCLA has beds."

"How do you know?"

"Because I know."

Janni comes into the office, escorted by Karen. She's still actively playing with Magical 61.

"Hey, Janni," Paul booms down to her.

"Hi," Janni answers. "Do you want to meet my friend, Magical 61?" If Janni notices Paul's face, she doesn't say anything. She doesn't seem afraid at all.

"Do you want to take a ride with us?" Paul asks.

Janni stops, suddenly showing concern. "Can Magical 61 come, too?"

"If she doesn't mind squeezing in the back with you and me," Maria answers.

"She doesn't."

"Okay, then."

Outside, I see their car. It looks like an unmarked police car, with a barrier between the front seat and the back.

"Janni, I'll be right behind you," I call as Janni gets in, followed by Maria.

·   ·   ·

THE ER HAS moved since we were here last April. The new Ronald Reagan UCLA Medical Center has opened. From the outside, it looks like a Hyatt hotel, not a hospital. I spot Maria and Paul's car.

I leave my car in the valet line, not bothering to take a ticket. If somebody wants to steal it, they can. I'm beyond caring.

I rush into the ER waiting room, expecting they'll already be back inside the ER.

"This way," I hear Paul call out from the waiting room.

"What's going on?" I ask.

"Waiting."

This makes no sense. I look over at the triage station. An old woman in a wheelchair is complaining she's been waiting for hours. The triage nurse is trying to placate her, along with an ER rep.

"January?" the triage nurse calls.

Janni screams. "I'm not January!" She starts hitting the triage nurse.

"Janni . . ." I try to intervene, but Janni is hitting her continuously.

Paul grabs her in his arms and picks her up. "We need to get her back," he says.

The nurse is so shocked she can barely nod. "Okay."

Paul carries Janni, who's hitting and kicking him. He doesn't react. I bring up the rear. The nurse leads us through the ER. I keep expecting her to turn into a room, but we keep walking, deeper and deeper into the ER, all the way to the very end, to the last room, which we enter.

Inside are two smaller rooms. As I pass the first, I see a man lying on the bed with a handcuff on his wrist, attached to the bed.

"This will be her room," the nurse says as we enter the second room, next door. Paul puts Janni down and she bolts.

"Hold on, Janni." He gently brings her back. "Let's sit on the bed."

The room is bare except for the bed. No EKG machine. No

automatic blood pressure machine. I realize we are in one of the rooms reserved for psychiatric patients. Everything is gone so the patients can't harm themselves or the staff.

"If you need anything, the nurse's call button is right there on the wall." The nurse looks at Paul. "Should I close the door?"

"Probably a good idea," he replies.

The nurse closes the door and it is just the four of us.

Maria comes up to me. "We need to go."

What?

"But she's not up to the unit yet," I protest. I'd expected them to stay with Janni and me through the whole process and explain why she needed to be an inpatient.

"That could take hours and we need to go."

Maria's phone's been ringing constantly. I know others are out there in the city who need them, but I need them, too.

"Don't you need to talk to the doctor?" I stammer.

"The nurse has my report."

I'm terrified. We've been here before and Janni didn't get admitted. I need them to make sure it happens this time.

"Please," I beg. "Don't go."

Maria puts her hand on my shoulder. "It'll be okay. I promise."

Paul takes his hand off Janni's shoulder. "Okay, Janni, you be good for your dad, okay?"

"Okay," she answers, strangely calm, but I'm still panicking as they turn to leave.

"Take care, okay?" Maria says to me.

And they're gone.

THERE ARE NO windows in here. I have no sense of time. I want to talk to Susan, but my phone isn't getting reception. I feel alone. Janni is physically here, but mentally miles away.

In the next room, the man handcuffed to his bed is now awake and screaming obscenities.

"Fuck you all . . . you fucking bitches! I know what you're fucking doing! You're playing with my cock! You fucking whores!"

I flinch at every word. I look at Janni dancing around, lost in her own world, playing with Magical 61. For the first time, I'm grateful for that world because it's protecting her from this one.

It's been six hours. Janni may be oblivious to the steady stream of obscenities coming from the next room, but I'm terrified. I feel like we have finally descended into the deepest reaches of hell. This was a mistake. I want to take her home. I want her safe in her bed, holding her stuffed bear, Hero.

Right outside these rooms is the security station. I walk out of Janni's room and up to one of the guards.

"We've been waiting hours for a psych consult."

"Sometimes it takes that long," he answers languidly. He must go through this every day. But I have to get out of here. There is no humanity in here and I feel mine slipping away.

"We're leaving. I am taking my daughter and leaving. I'm not going to stay and let her be exposed to all this."

"You can't leave," the guard tells me, standing up, at least a foot taller than I am.

I look up at him, shocked. "Of course we can leave. You can't keep us here! We came here voluntarily!"

"Maybe you did," he answers, "but she has a hold."

A hold? This has never happened to us before. "For how long?"

"Until the doctor sees her, then maybe she can go."

"So we just have to wait?"

The security guard sits back down. "Yep."

I finally realize what has happened. Maria and Paul 5150'd her, placed her on an involuntary hold. That was how they got her into UCLA. The standard hold is three days.

Janni snaps back to reality for a moment as I reenter her room. "Are we leaving?"

I look at her. What have I done? Why didn't I just take her home? "Not yet."

"I'm hungry," Janni whines.

I turn back to the security guard. "I want to see the damn doctor!" I'm losing control. I want to go home.

"The doctor is coming," the guard answers placidly.

I turn back to Janni. "Janni, stay here. I'll be right back." I don't want to leave her alone in this place, but I have no choice.

I charge through the nurses' station, scanning for the ER doctor who did the medical check on Janni when we first arrived.

I find him, leaning up against the station, chatting to another doctor.

"Where is the psychiatrist?" I yell at his back.

He turns to me. "I just called. They're pretty busy."

"My daughter is in that room next to a guy handcuffed to his bed, swearing obscenities."

"I understand—"

"No, you don't understand!" I cut him off. "Nobody fucking understands! This is my six-year-old daughter I brought here for help, and she's not getting any! It isn't your child, so what do you care?! None of you give a flying fuck!" I am screaming, my breath heaving, on the verge of breaking down. I want to break down. I want them to drag me away. But I can't. Janni needs me.

The ER goes deathly quiet. I feel every eye that is awake on me. The ER doctor remains stone-faced.

"I do understand," he says quietly. "I can see how much you love your daughter and want to help her, but what you're doing right now isn't helping. She needs you to stay calm."

"Being calm hasn't gotten her any help!" I shout back.

"All you're doing right now is scaring other patients."

I open my mouth, but nothing comes out. I fight tears in the corner of my eyes. I'm cracking.

"I'm sorry." I sniffle. "I'm just scared."

He nods. "I will page the psychiatrist again."

I nod, wiping my eyes. "She's hungry. I need to get her food. Where's the cafeteria?"

He takes me gently by the arm and points down the hall.

"Through those doors and to the right." He looks at me. "You gotta hang in there. Be strong for her. It's gonna be okay."

I nod. I don't believe him, just like I didn't believe Maria, but I still want him to keep telling me it's going to be okay.

I DON'T KNOW what Janni will eat. They have grilled cheese and she eats that, but not all the time. I buy several things, hoping something will appeal to her. Grilled cheese, onion rings, corn, rice. I bring everything back and show them off. She picks at the onion rings.

A young man sticks his head in the door and looks down at his chart. "Is this January?"

"Not January!" Janni screams, her eyes down, focused on the onion rings.

"Sorry," he apologizes. "I'm the psychiatric fellow," he says to me, although he looks more like he's going out to a nightclub. I give him Janni's history. I cover everything since she was born. I don't know if it matters anymore.

He nods, taking notes. "Okay, Janni. Can I talk to you for a minute?"

"Do you want to see my pet rat?" Janni holds out her empty palm.

"I'll go outside," I tell him. I don't want to run the risk he might think I am influencing her. He needs to see what we see every day. I pray he does.

Five minutes later he comes out, still writing in his notes.

"So what do you think?"

"Well . . . ," he begins. My heart sinks. He doesn't see it. Janni's not being violent at this very moment. She just seems "imaginative." I resign myself to the fact we came for nothing. At least she'll get to sleep in her own bed tonight. That is all I want to do now. Just sleep.

"She's definitely saying some odd things. She is pretty obsessed with this world of hers. She told me all about the animals and girls who live there. 'Calalini,' I think she called it."

"Are you going to admit her?"

"Let me go talk to my supervisor and see what he has to say and I'll come back."

"How long?"

"Soon."

"Soon" is ninety minutes later. He returns with a piece of paper.

"What's this?" I ask.

"This is the authorization to treat."

"So you are admitting her?"

"Yeah, we're going to admit her. She said some things that were a little concerning."

It is all I can do to stand up. I can barely believe it.

It's over. I've done it. I've gotten her into UCLA. Everything is going to be okay now. They will figure out how to help her.

CHAPTER TWENTY-NINE

February 2009

WARNING: REMOVE ALL METAL FROM YOUR PERSON.

I look down at my wedding ring. It's gold, a metal totally impervious to the effects of magnets. I remember buying it nine years ago. It wasn't expensive. Susan and I went together to pick out our rings at the Sears jewelry counter. It wasn't romantic, but it was fun because we did it together. We used to do everything together. Susan was my partner, my best friend. Now it feels like we never knew each other before Janni. We're soldiers on a battlefield now, a new relationship forged from being in a common crisis, a war against the still officially unnamed enemy inside Janni.

I take off my ring and put it inside the locker anyway. Soldiers going into a battle they fear they may not return from also remove their personal effects, keeping only their dog tags. Every day I feel like I am going deeper and deeper into a place I will never come back from.

My dog tag is not around my neck, but sitting in a wheelchair as I enter the MRI room. Janni is my dog tag, my identification.

"I don't want to do it," she tells me.

I sigh. It's after 11 P.M. and I've been at UCLA since visiting hours began at 7 P.M., waiting for Radiology to take her in for an MRI. If anyone can get her through this, it's me, and I have to get her through this because tonight could reveal this enemy I've been fighting for more than a year. If I can see it, then I can conquer it.

"It doesn't hurt, Janni. It's just loud. The noise makes it scary."

"I don't want to do it."

"We have earplugs." The radiology technician pulls them out of his ears. "Like this."

They're the little foam ones you roll up and stick inside your ear. I know them well. I tried them a year ago, along with headphones, hoping the combination would completely block out the sound of Bodhi's crying.

"She won't wear those," I say.

"That's all we have," the technician says to me.

"I don't want to do it," Janni says.

I squat down next to her. "Janni, we need to see what's going on inside your brain." My voice is calm, but I'm begging. *I need this, Janni. I need to see the "enemy."*

"No."

"We can have the doctor order a sedative," Gillian offers. Gillian is a nurse from the child psych unit who must be with Janni anytime she is off the unit.

But then it won't happen tonight. Her doctor's gone home, and we're just a few feet from the machine that can turn a light on in the darkness we've been living in for so long. I turn back to Janni. I have to convince her to get into the machine.

"Janni, what if I go to the car and get your headphones?"

"We have headphones," the radiology tech says.

"What?"

"We have headphones." He goes to a drawer and retrieves a set of headphones.

The question of why he didn't tell me this before annoys me.

"See, Janni, they have headphones."

"Can I get music?" Janni asks, spotting a long cord running out of the headphones.

"Can you pipe in music through this cord?" I ask the tech.

"No music. Sorry. The cord is so we can talk to the patient inside the machine."

Dammit, I think. The headphones will only dull the sound of the MRI, not eliminate it. She needs something to distract her mind from the noise in the tunnel.

"Janni, I'll sing to you. I'll sing so loud you won't be able to hear the machine." I look down at Janni, desperate.

Janni is silent for a moment, then looks up at me. "What will you sing?"

"Anything you want. What about 'Yellow Submarine'?"

Susan bought me The Beatles' *1* album for an anniversary gift a few years ago. I never thought I'd be able to listen to it in the car, but one day I tried and Janni started singing along.

Try to see it my way,
Only time will tell if I am right or I am wrong . . .

Those moments gave me hope.

I can see Janni thinking.

"We can work it out," I say, smiling.

She smiles and rubs her hands together, getting the reference.

The tech helps her onto the MRI table, but as soon as he starts to strap her down, she sits back up again.

"Sweetie," the tech tells her. "I'm sorry I have to do this, but if you move, we won't get good pictures."

"Janni, it's okay," I take her hand. "Just lie down."

I watch as the tech immobilizes her head with tape.

Janni cries. I can count on one hand the number of times I've seen real tears come from her eyes.

"It's gonna be okay, Janni," I say. "Daddy's here." I take her hand in mine.

The tech inserts a mirror in front of her face. "This is so you can see your daddy." He turns to me. "We ready?"

I nod.

He disappears into the control room. A few seconds later, I hear him over the PA: "Okay, here we go."

The table slides back into the tunnel, and Janni begins whimpering like a lost dog.

"It's okay, Janni. Daddy's right here. Can you see me?" I wave to her face in the mirror.

"Yes," she says in a childlike tone I'm not used to hearing. The table retreats into the tunnel, designed more for an adult. Her hand, still holding mine, disappears inside the tunnel, but I keep holding on as my arm is swallowed up. My shoulder hits the outside of the tunnel, but I won't let go. I hunker down, putting my head inside the tunnel with Janni, following her in.

My feet leave the floor as the table pulls me in, then stops. My entire upper body is inside the tunnel. I prop myself up over Janni's legs, lifting my head high so Janni sees me in the mirror.

She is still whimpering.

"It's like a den in here," I say, my voice echoing inside the tunnel. "It's like we're prairie dogs. Remember the prairie dogs we used to see when I took you to the zoo? This is like what prairie dogs live in." I yip like a prairie dog.

"Okay, starting up," the tech calls over the PA. The machine starts to wind up like a jet engine. Despite the noise, I still hear Janni's crying. I could probably hear her over a class-five hurricane after being so wired to her crying from when she was a baby, six years ago.

"Janni, it's okay. Look at me, Janni. Look in the mirror."

I see her eyes move in the mirror and locate me. Her head is immobilized so the techs can get clear images of her brain.

"Can you see me?" I wave in the cramped space.

"I can see you."

"Keep your eyes on me, Janni. Keep watching me. Don't pay attention to anything but me. I will explain everything. That noise is the sound of a giant magnet spinning around you. This magnet makes the ions in your body align with the . . ." I stop, seeing her mouth open in a full cry.

What the fuck am I doing? I'm still trying to teach her, even now. I suppose it is the last remnant of my belief that all of this is just the result of her genius. But she doesn't need a teacher. She needs her dad.

"Janni! Janni! Look in the mirror! Keep your eyes on Daddy!" I see her look at me in the mirror. Our eyes meet. I start to sing:

> *"In the town where I was born,*
> *Lived a man, who sailed to sea.*
> *And he told us of his life*
> *In the Land of Submarines."*

The machine gets louder. "Okay, starting imaging." The tech's voice comes over the PA. "Hold still now."

The machine starts clicking loudly.

Janni cries out.

"Janni!" I shout over the loud clicking of the machine. "Keep your eyes on me!"

She looks back in the mirror at me.

"So we sailed into the sun,
till we found the sea of green.
And we lived beneath the waves,
In our yellow submarine . . ."

Every time the machine gets louder, so does my singing, until I'm shouting at the top of my lungs.

"And our friends are all aboard,
many more of them live next door . . ."

The clicks alternate with loud booms. Every time I see Janni look away, I call her back to the mirror. She does and I resume singing, screaming the lyrics now.

"As we live a life of ease;
Every one of us has all we need"

"All we need!" I shout, waving my free arm and jerking my head inside the machine. I feel like we're rewinding in time, back to the ball pit at IKEA when she was a baby, when I got in with her and jumped around, not caring what anybody thought because it made her laugh.

"Sky of Blue! *Sky of Blue!* And Sea of Green! *Sea of Green!*" I'm like a drunk at a karaoke bar. "In our yellow, *in our yellow* . . . submarine, *submarine! Ah-hah!*"

Janni smiles at me through the mirror.

"We all live in a yellow submarine, yellow submarine,
yellow submarine.
We all live in a yellow submarine, a yellow submarine,
a yellow submarine."

I run through every song I know the lyrics to, never taking my eyes off her. She is looking away more often now. I can see her mouth opening in a cry made silent by the roar of the machine.

This is taking too long. She's trying to twist her head. I need to do something quickly or she will go into a panic.

"*I am January Paige,*" I shout, remembering the song Susan and I made up for her when she was a baby. I see her stop moving and focus on me in the mirror.

"And this is my song.
If you do not sing to me,
I'll cry all night long."

She doesn't smile, but she doesn't look away, either. I pray that maybe, just maybe, she still remembers, and if she still remembers, then the enemy has not completely taken her from me yet.

CHAPTER THIRTY

March 2009

Janni's name has changed.

It is Jani now, with the second "n" deleted.

Here at UCLA, the kids get their names outside the door to their room, typed up in large, crazy fonts on the computer with an image of something they love, like a horse, a dog, or an action figure.

The first time Susan and I saw it, we thought it was a mistake, but a teenage girl who is on the wing with her is named Dani. Jani will talk to her about her rats and Dani doesn't bat an eye, eagerly listening to her stories of a world that only Jani can see. Dani seems to give her a sense of normalcy, like she had at Alhambra and Loma Linda.

Though we didn't argue, happy for her to go by any variation of the name we gave her years before, it was still sad for Susan and me. We knew contracting "Janni" from "January" didn't make as much sense, but it was our name for her, our special name for our special little girl. And now it is gone. And even though Susan and I never said a word about it to each other, I could tell we both felt the same thing: that her name change was like cutting the umbilical cord.

IT'S BEEN ABOUT a month since Jani's been at UCLA and we're at our Family Meeting, grateful to be part of the "treatment team," which includes Jani's doctor, Dr. Kim, a young Asian-American woman, and Georgia, our social worker, who's nearing retirement age. Dr. Kim is Jani's primary psychiatrist, but in reality the entire Resnick Neuropsychiatric Hospital at UCLA is working on Jani, including the head psychiatrist, Dr. DeAntonio. Kim's job, along with consulting with Dr. Howe (making her the first inpatient doctor to do that), is to fight with the insurance company to allow Jani treatment as long as she needs it.

"She is a difficult case," Georgia starts off. "If it were thirty or forty years ago, she'd be in the back ward of Camarillo State Hospital."

Susan jumps in. "So there were kids like Jani. What happened to them?"

"Well, obviously I wasn't able to follow up on them through their lives, but most got better over time with the right medication," Georgia responds. "But we don't have that kind of time anymore. Patients used to have six months to a year inpatient, but nowadays, insurance companies don't pay."

Two weeks into Jani's stay here we got a letter from Blue Shield saying they were stopping payment. The only reason Jani is still here at UCLA is because in my desperate attempts to continue her care, I found this state agency, the Department of Managed Care, that overturned Blue Shield's decision, even going so far as to express disgust that the HMO would consider discharging a child "so obviously unstable." Under California state law, the decision of the Department of

Managed Care's doctor was final and could not be appealed, so Blue Shield had no choice but to start paying again. But the law doesn't say *how long* Blue Shield has to keep paying. They sent us a letter initially authorizing only another three days, at which time they would "review" Jani's case again. "Review," we have learned, is a euphemism for "not going to pay anymore." Blue Shield will keep trying to have her discharged and I will keep fighting them.

"I'm sorry it's taken so long to get the results of the MRI," Dr. Kim tells us, looking up from her folder of notes, "but I was waiting for the images to be analyzed by a neurologist before I got back to you."

Susan and I wait nervously.

"For the most part, everything was normal," Kim continues. "There was one bright spot in her thalamus, which is what I wanted to get analyzed."

"What does that mean?" I ask.

"Well, usually in scans of the brain, areas that are ischemic, oxygen deprived," she gestures, "show up very bright."

"And that's not something to be concerned about?" I press.

"It doesn't impair her function," Kim replies.

"You don't think that is the cause of her behavior?" Susan asks.

Kim shakes her head. "We talked about it in rounds. It's a very tiny part of the thalamus believed to be the primary center through which neurological commands and signals are exchanged between the body and the brain. It's kind of like a switchboard."

"And you're sure this ischemic part of her thalamus wouldn't have any role at all?" I ask, desperate for answers. This is as far inside Jani's brain as we have ever gotten.

Dr. Kim shakes her head. "It's what we call a stressor on the brain, but no, it wouldn't be the cause. It's a type of stroke event, although obviously very mild. They often occur in the womb, during birth, or shortly thereafter."

I feel my blood vessels constrict and a sharp pain in my skull.

"What causes them?" I manage.

Kim shrugs. "We don't know. It could be a genetic predisposition or a random occurrence."

"What about shaking?" Susan asks, glancing sideways at me.

"I'm sorry?" Kim is confused, looking from Susan to me.

I lower my eyes. Sadly, after everything that has happened, the truth is I'd almost forgotten about that.

I exhale. "From the moment Jani was born, she never slept. Before we learned that nonstop stimulation helped her sleep, she would only sleep twenty or thirty minutes at a time, little power naps, getting a total of four to five hours a day. So we didn't sleep either. We'd been getting by because we would take Jani in shifts, five hours on and five hours off. Then Susan had to go back to work because we needed the money. I had her every night, all night, without a break, holding her while she screamed and screamed." I pause, remembering the fear in Jani's big blue eyes. "One night, I finally snapped and shook her, yelling, 'Why won't you sleep?!' She immediately started to cry and it shocked me out of it." I stop, struggling to find the words. "It is the worst thing I have ever done in my life. I wish I could take it back, but I can't. I did it."

I turn to Susan, trying to read her expression. I don't see hatred. I see doubt, her asking herself if all of this can be traced back to me. I don't know what to say. If I damaged Jani's brain, how do I make amends for that?

Susan holds my gaze for a moment, then turns back to Kim and Georgia. "I actually don't think he caused this. Jani was always different. Even in the womb she never slept. But what do you think?"

I look at Kim, who appears to be thinking. She takes a long time before she answers. "Well, there is no way to know for sure, but her crying right after . . . what he did, is actually a good sign. I would be more concerned if there was a reduced response."

"There was no change," Susan says. "I checked her out and we saw the doctor right after. We were always seeing her pediatrician because we were always trying to find out why she wasn't sleeping."

"So I might have damaged her thalamus?" I ask softly.

Kim shifts in her chair, clearly uncomfortable. "The thalamus is buried pretty deep in the brain, and it would likely take more than that to cause this ischemic event. Usually, it just happens. The blood vessels in that area never fully developed and when blood starts to flow, they burst." She pauses, then looks at me. "It doesn't cause schizophrenia. It's a stressor on the brain that could bring it on earlier, but it's not the cause."

"What about her hand movements?" Susan asks, referring to Jani's constant rolling of her wrists, at speeds so fast it must be painful, yet Jani shows no reaction. "Could the thalamus be causing that?"

Dr. Kim shakes her head. "It's not neurological, like a spasm. She doesn't do it constantly. We think it's more a form of stimming, like in autism."

Susan gives an exasperated sigh. "Great, so we're going back to autism again."

"We don't think she has autism," Dr. Kim answers almost meekly. "We've talked about that because many of the doctors here are experts in that area. They don't feel she fits the profile because the two dominant symptoms Jani shows are her preference for and interaction with her invisible friends and her corresponding aggression toward real people. Children with autism get set off by things the rest of us are aware of but which don't bother us to the same extent. We don't know what sets Jani off."

"So what is it, then?" Susan demands.

"It's still early," Kim replies. She looks up and clears her throat, "but I can tell you that at this point we've ruled out everything but child-onset schizophrenia."

The room is suddenly so silent I can hear my own blood surging past my eardrums. I sit back and look at Susan, who looks at me.

It's not a shock. Susan always suspected Jani had schizophrenia, but I wanted to deny it. I wanted something that could be fixed. Schizophrenia cannot be fixed. There is no cure.

Even after everything that has happened and what people said along the way, I still held out hope. I pushed Dr. Howe to admit it was schizophrenia not because I wanted that to be the real diagnosis but because her reluctance gave me hope. Now that Kim has actually said it, the reality hits home.

My mind shifts to what life is like for schizophrenics, and it terrifies me.

Jani will probably never be able to go to school, let alone college. She'll never have a boyfriend or get married. I think sadly of how other fathers used to tell me, in reference to how pretty she was, "When she grows up, you're gonna need a shotgun!" No, I won't, I realize.

I look down at Bodhi. He will never have a normal big sister. I wanted to believe that one day Jani would snap out of this and finally love him like I always wanted her to. Now I realize she won't, because she can't. How she treats him now is how she'll treat him for the rest of his life. When Susan and I are dead and gone, he'll be taking care of her, still taking her abuse. That is his future.

I start to cry. I hear a low moan escape from Susan, followed by a sob. She grabs my arm. I put my hand over hers and turn back to Kim, wiping the tears away with my free hand. I push down my pain. I have to focus. I have to plan the rest of Jani's life now.

"So it is schizophrenia, then?" I say.

Dr. Kim looks so sad, like she wants to cry with Susan. I watch her struggling to be a professional, but she can't quite do it.

"Um," she begins, looking so much like a girl in high school, not an MD and PhD from UCLA, "in order to make the diagnosis official, we need more time. Typically, we need to see the symptoms over a six-month period. But given that we have her history from Dr. Howe, I suspect we'll be able to make a definitive diagnosis before that."

Susan is still crying and unable to speak. I can barely speak. My anguish wants to be released, but I have to push it down so I can focus. Questions must be asked and answered.

"What is her prognosis?"

Kim looks down again before looking up to meet my eyes.

"Well, the fact that she is so resistant to medication is not good," she says, "but she's very intelligent. I would say . . . fifty-fifty. She has a fifty percent chance of getting better and a fifty percent chance of getting worse." She pauses. "I wish I could give you better odds."

It's hard to breathe. "I appreciate you being honest with us."

"Always," Kim answers, looking down again.

Georgia leans across the table, putting her hand out, taking mine and Susan's in hers.

"The important thing to remember now is not to give up."

"That's right," Kim adds. "We're not giving up. Jani has responded well when she had to receive a PRN of Thorazine. Our plan right now, assuming you approve, of course, is to start Thorazine as a standard. It's not something we generally do, but given the severity of Jani's case we feel it is warranted."

"This is not the end of the world," Georgia says. "It is our job to treat Jani. Your job is to make sure you both will be okay."

I shake my head. "She's already been through so many medications, and none of them work perfectly."

Kim and Georgia exchange looks. "No," Kim answers, "but new medications are coming on the market all the time."

"That is why you have to be strong," Georgia adds. "Don't give up."

"We won't," Susan speaks up. "We can't. She's our daughter and we love her."

"And honestly," Dr. Kim replies, "that is why I actually do have hope for her. She has the two of you."

"We're not giving up," I answer. I clear my throat for the question I really need to know. "I'm no doctor, but most schizophrenics I've seen are scared of their hallucinations."

Kim nods slowly. "The disease presents differently in everyone, but generally that is true."

"Jani's not afraid of her hallucinations. They're her friends, even the ones who bite her and scratch her, like 400."

Kim nods again. "That's a good thing, though. I'm sure you wouldn't want her living in terror."

"No. No, I wouldn't." I struggle to say what I have to say. "But they are very appealing to her, more than anything in this world. What if . . . one day she goes into her world and just doesn't come back?"

Kim appears taken back.

"Is there a possibility," I continue, "that this is catatonic schizophrenia?"

Kim looks to Georgia, seemingly for reassurance.

"I mean, that is a version of schizophrenia, right? What if she has that?"

Kim regains her professional demeanor. "Well, first of all, there is not complete agreement that catatonic schizophrenia exists. Patients definitely go into their own fantasy world, but I have never seen anybody fail to come back. If that is what you are worried about, I wouldn't be concerned."

But that is exactly what I am worried about. We are through the looking glass now. Things that I thought could never happen have happened. Kim can tell me until she is blue in the face that Jani will never just slip away into Calilini, but what if she does?

CHAPTER THIRTY-ONE

Late March 2009

W hat food did you bring?" Jani asks me as I enter the unit.
"I brought mac 'n' cheese from Burger King . . ." I stop,
seeing Jani's middle finger, splinted, wrapped in bandages.

"What happened to your finger?"

"Adam slammed my finger in the door. Look." She removes the
bandages. Her finger is mottled black and blue.

Adam is another boy on the unit. He's a year younger than Jani,
but he's the first child on the unit who's worse than she is.

I immediately get a nurse.

"We had it checked by a doctor and x-rayed," she tells me. "It's
not broken."

"What happened?"

"She called him a dog; he hit her and she hit him back."

Oh no. Jani calls all people "dogs," but this kid is African-American
and he may have had a bad experience with the word. Is this going to

be Jani's future, I wonder, unintentionally starting fights because she doesn't understand social cues?

I go back to her room, where she's eating the Burger King food I brought.

I left the door open and a small boy appears at the door.

"That's Adam," Jani tells me.

Adam, a smile on his face, the same twisted smile I've seen on Jani's face, takes a step into her room, a violation of the rules. He is now trying to provoke her.

Jani moves toward him, lifting her arm in preparation to hit. I grab her by her shirt and hold her back just as a male nurse, Adam's assigned "one-to-one," reaches the door and pulls Adam back.

"Sorry," the nurse says. "He got away from me for a minute." He closes the door.

Jani immediately pushes it open again.

"Jani, where are you going?" I ask nervously, even though I can guess. "Come back and finish your food."

"I have to hit him," she tells me in the same voice she used going after Honey.

I run out into the hall. Jani is already at the entrance to Adam's room. She disappears inside. I race in and see her with her arm raised, moving in for the strike.

Adam is struggling to get free of the nurse holding him. I grab on to Jani and start moving backward, pulling her along with me. The nurse and I look like boxing referees trying to keep two fighters apart.

"I need to hit him," Jani repeats.

"No, you don't."

"He hurt me."

"That's because you called him a dog. He didn't like that. You have to call people by their names."

Jani is struggling against me. "Let me hit him!"

"I need something to distract her," I call to another nurse in the day room, the unit's communal area, and look around. At the end of the corridor is another room. This one is filled with musical instruments, including a drum set. Maybe I can get her banging on the drums as a way to vent her aggression.

"Could we get the music room opened?"

The nurse unlocks the music room.

I take the drumsticks and pound on the snare and the floor tom.

"Here." I hand Jani the drumsticks, and she hits the floor tom without much enthusiasm.

I pick up a second set of sticks. "No, like this." I pound the hell out of the floor tom, the snare drum, and the crash cymbals. "Really hit 'em," I yell over my noise. "This is something you can hit. It's okay because it's not alive. Really get into it! Take your aggression out! Beat the heck out of them! It's okay."

Jani hits harder.

Adam appears at the door, followed by his nurse.

"Sorry," the nurse says apologetically, trying to pull Adam away. "He heard the drums."

"I want to play, too!" Adam calls into the room.

"You can't right now. Jani is in there," the nurse answers, trying to steer Adam away.

"It's okay," I call to the nurse. "He can come in. There are two sets of sticks."

The nurse looks at me like I'm crazy.

"Are you sure?"

If Jani is ever going to be able to survive in the outside world, she has to learn how to deal with people. If she can socialize with Adam, despite wanting to hit him, then that would be a huge breakthrough.

"Yeah," I reply. "There's enough drums for everybody." I flip my sticks, holding them out to Adam.

"But first let's make sure everybody understands the rules. The only thing you can hit with the sticks are the drums. There will be no hitting of each other. Understood?"

Adam nods. I hand him the sticks and position him on the opposite side of the kit from Jani.

"Adam, you hit this drum, which is called the floor tom, and Jani, you hit this drum, which is called the snare drum."

Adam bangs on the floor tom.

"I don't want to play anymore," Jani says, tossing her sticks on the floor.

I pick them up and hold them out to her.

"No, I am going to teach you and Adam how to play the drums." I know I am tempting fate by having them within an arm's reach of each other with wooden drumsticks, but I am determined to make this work.

Jani takes the sticks, bangs on the snare a few times, then reaches for Adam with her right stick.

"No," I say, grabbing her arm. "We hit drums, not people. Come on, you two. Let's see if we can get a beat going."

Jani goes back to drumming. Adam is beating the skins as well. They are completely out of time with each other, but I don't care. If I can get them to play beside each other without hitting, I've succeeded.

I see Jani extend her arm again, past the crash cymbal, drumstick raised above Adam's head.

"No!" I say, grabbing her arm again. "Jani, if you hit Adam, then we have to leave the music room."

Jani pulls back her arm and screams, hitting the drumstick against the side of her head with full force.

I am so shocked I can't move. Jani screams again and pounds the stick into the side of her head as hard as she can.

The need for action finally breaks through the shock of what I'm seeing, and I jump forward, wrenching the drumstick from her hand.

She uses the other stick to hit her head, and I quickly take that as well, standing there, breathing heavily.

"Jani! Why did you do that?" I want an answer. I need an answer. Hitting herself like that must hurt beyond belief, yet she is not responding to the pain.

Jani suddenly looks up at me as if she just realized I am here. She looks scared and confused, like she isn't sure what just happened.

Oh, my God.

For more than a year, I've wanted to see the enemy and I just saw it. That wasn't a behavior. Something took control of Jani's body, and when it was gone, Jani was left with no idea what had happened. Up until now, there was still a small part of me that wondered if she could control this, but there is no doubt anymore. Its name is schizophrenia, and if she doesn't do what it wants, it will turn on her, making her hurt herself.

CHAPTER THIRTY-TWO

Early April 2009

Visiting hours at UCLA are longer on the weekends, from 2 to 4 P.M., the only time all three of us go to visit Jani. It's our family time, but there is one other reason we bring Bodhi. He is a necessary guinea pig. The only way to know if the medications are working is if we can make it through the entire two hours without Jani attempting to hurt Bodhi.

"Bodhi!" Jani cries and runs up to his stroller as we come in. She is happy to see him, and that is an encouraging sign, but I don't start jumping for joy. We still have two hours to get through.

"Hi, Bodhi." She looks down, waiting, like she's expecting an answer. I think she's hoping he'll understand her and be the flesh-and-blood friend she's never had.

Susan lies down on Jani's bed, like she always does. These trips to UCLA really seem to exhaust her. She talks to Jani, asking her about the other kids on the unit, particularly if there are any other girls, and if she ever plays with any of them.

I take Bodhi out of his stroller, and he begins crawling around the room. For the life of me, I can't remember when he started to crawl. He's already pulling himself up to a standing position, using the chair next to Jani's desk to reach for the painted bobblehead animals Jani makes in occupational therapy.

I watch him get his stubby fingers around a bobblehead dog. I glance over at Jani, who is still talking to Susan, praying she won't notice.

But she does. I wince as she moves to him, grabbing the dog away.

"Bodhi, no!" she scolds him like a puppy that just peed on the floor. But she doesn't hit him. She just holds the toy, looking down at him, telling him he can't touch her things. At least she didn't hit him. Maybe the Thorazine is having an effect.

Bodhi starts to cry, not understanding why he can't have the dog.

"Jani," I say to her, "let him have it. He just wants to look at it."

"No." She lifts the dog high above her head so Bodhi can't reach it.

"Jani, he just wants to explore. That's how babies learn about the world around them, by touch."

"But he'll teethe on them," she complains.

That is true. Bodhi puts everything in his mouth.

"But that's just part of the exploration. His mouth is more sensitive than his hands are at this age."

"I don't want baby slobber on them." She scoops up all her toys in her arms.

"We can wash them off."

"He'll break them," she argues.

"How?"

"With his teeth."

"Jani, your toys are solid plastic. That's the whole reason plastic was invented. It's unbreakable. Humans can't bite through plastic. It's impossible."

"Bodhi can."

"No, he can't."

"Yes, he can," she says, convinced, even though she's never seen him do it.

I take one of her toys, a Littlest Pet Shop dog, from her hands and put it in my mouth. I bite down as hard as I can and pull it out.

"See?" I show her. "Not even any teeth marks. And my teeth are way stronger than Bodhi's."

Jani is still jealously guarding her toys. "I still don't want him teething on my stuff."

"How come I can put your toys in my mouth but Bodhi can't?"

"Because you're not going to break them."

"Jani," I say, fighting a sense of exasperation. "I just showed you nobody can bite through plastic!"

"He will." Jani looks at Bodhi like he isn't human.

There is no reasoning with her. I can see it in her eyes. She really believes Bodhi can bite through her toys.

"Fine. Then you need to put your toys where he can't reach them."

I bring his toy cars out from under his stroller. "Here, Bodhi. Come play with me."

Bodhi needs someone who'll be kind to him. Susan and I bring him here every weekend, to the sister who is supposed to love him. But she can't, I remind myself. The schizophrenia won't let her.

Because Susan is lying there, Bodhi crawls over to Jani's bed and pulls himself up. He finds one of Jani's stuffed animals, a dog, and moves it to his mouth. He chews on one of its legs, probably because it feels good on his gums.

"Bodhi!" Jani moves like lightning, snatching the dog from Bodhi's mouth so hard I am afraid she'll pull his teeth with it.

I grab the dog and put the same leg in my mouth and chew, then hand it back to Jani.

"See? It was me," I lie.

Last weekend, Bodhi knocked one of her toys over. She didn't see it happen but heard it. When she turned and saw her toy on the floor, she started moving toward Bodhi, fist up, but I was able intervene.

"Jani, Bodhi didn't do it," I said, desperate to protect Bodhi without having to leave.

And then an idea came into my head. If Jani's grasp on reality was basically gone, maybe I could make her believe something that didn't happen.

"Jani, didn't you feel that earthquake just now?" I asked, testing my theory. Of course, I was hoping she would say no and wonder why I was asking, but instead she looked confused for a moment.

"Yes," she finally answered.

I swallowed down my sense of devastation. "That's right. The earthquake knocked over your toy." I lied to protect my son. And she believed me.

Now I am biting down on the stuffed dog again. "See? It was me."

"No, it wasn't. It was Bodhi," she says now.

I deflate. It isn't working this time because she actually saw his teeth on her stuffed animal. I prepare to stop her from hitting him.

But she grabs the stuffed dog, turns away, and opens the bathroom door in her room.

"Don't forget to wipe yourself and then flush the toilet and wash your hands," Susan calls out.

I hear water run.

Suddenly, Jani emerges from the bathroom, wailing and in tears.

"Jani, what is it?" I rush to her.

She holds up the stuffed dog. "He's all wet."

The dog is soaked.

"I was trying to wash the baby slobber off," she continues through her tears, "but he got all wet!"

I force a laugh, hoping I can prevent her from going off by playing down what happened.

"That's no big deal. We can just pop him in the dryer. He'll be fine."

"No, we can't! He's ruined. I'll have to throw him away." She drops the dog into the trash. "Bye, bye, doggie."

"Jani . . ." I retrieve the dog from the trash. "Actually, he'll probably dry in the sun."

Out of the corner of my eye, I see Jani striding for Bodhi. Susan sits up like a gunshot, and I break for the other side of the room; as wired as we are, we are still too slow. Jani hits Bodhi square in the back, hard.

I reach out and pull her back, angry because my reflexes are slipping. I guess more than a year of always being ready to react has worn me out.

"Jani, it's okay," I say to her, soothingly. "We can dry him."

She turns and starts hitting me.

I get down on my knees, my hands on her shoulders, trying to reach her.

"Jani, we can dry him—" I break off as she hits me in the face.

I suck in my breath, tasting blood from my lip.

Susan takes Bodhi out. She has gone to get the nursing staff, to tell them what happened, that the meds aren't working.

A nurse enters.

"Jani, what's going on?" She sees Jani hitting me. "Whoa, Jani, that is not okay!"

"Bodhi put her stuffed dog in his mouth, and then she tried to wash it off but got it all wet," I calmly explain to the nurse through Jani's blows. "I keep telling her we can dry it, but she won't believe me."

The nurse puts her hands on her hips and sternly says, "Jani, you need to calm down or your parents are going to have to leave."

This pisses me off. I'm not leaving while Jani is like this. Jani turns and hits the nurse, who puts out her hands and grabs Jani's wrists.

"Jani, that is not okay!"

Jani screams and drops to the floor, her arms and legs striking out in all directions. I have seen her do this before. As long as you don't get within range, you don't get hurt. I desperately want to believe that this is her way of trying *not* to hurt the people around her.

Of course, rather than standing back like Jani wants us to, the nurse moves in, trying to restrain Jani, and gets kicked in the side of her head.

"Okay," the nurse says, trying to hold down Jani's legs. "That's it. Your family has to leave."

"Good!" Jani cries back. "I want them to go!"

I am stunned.

I get down on my knees, within range of her blows, but I don't care.

"Jani, you don't really mean that," I tell her, afraid this is the beginning of her choosing Calilini and institutionalization over us, over me.

"Yes, I do!" she screams back. "I want you to go!"

"Jani, that is the schizophrenia talking, not you."

"It is me!" Jani yells and twists, driving her foot into my chest. I grunt, but hold my ground.

"Jani, I'm not leaving. I don't care how hard you hit me. I won't leave." I want Jani to know that there's nothing she can do to drive me away. I will never give up. But I am also talking to the schizophrenia, reminding it that I am not about to let it take Jani without a fight.

"I want you to go away!" Jani roars.

"I'm not leaving," I repeat, with a calmness I don't feel.

Jani gives her earsplitting scream.

I hear Bodhi crying and look up.

Susan is standing at the door with Bodhi in her arms.

"Get Bodhi off the unit!" I yell at her.

"No."

"I don't want him to see this!"

"She's my daughter, too, you know!" she retorts. "Why don't *you* take Bodhi and *I'll* stay with Jani?"

I stare at her while Jani pogos her legs into my stomach. "Get him out of here. This is no life for a baby."

Susan hesitates. I know she doesn't want to go, but she needs to. We can't keep exposing Bodhi to Jani's illness. But that is not the only reason I want Susan to take Bodhi. I feel possessive of Jani. She is my responsibility. I'm the only one who has the ability to go deep into her world, as far as she goes. She is still going, and I am still going with her.

CHAPTER THIRTY-THREE

Mid-April 2009

When I arrive at UCLA, Jani is lying in the middle of the corridor, staring up at the lights in the ceiling.

I lie down next to her. "Jani?"

She doesn't answer but instead continues staring up at the lights.

I put my face above hers and turn to look up. Unable to stare into the lights anymore, I turn back to Jani. She disappears into the two dark spots in my vision.

When I can see Jani clearly again, I see that her pupils are fully dilated, despite the fact that she is staring into bright lights. No drug did this. Whatever she is seeing is not the lights.

"Jani, what's up there?" I ask.

"Flying dogs," Jani answers flatly.

I debate if there is any point in telling her dogs can't fly.

"Dogs can't fly, Jani." I decide to confront her with this reality because I'm not willing to let her go without a fight. "They don't have

wings and their bones aren't hollow. That's what makes birds light
enough to achieve lift." I am still trying to reach her the only way I
know how: by teaching her.

"These ones can."

"What kind of dogs are they?" I ask.

"Golden retrievers."

The doctors here told us they believe Jani has probably always
experienced hallucinations, which is why she never reacted to them
with fear. If you grew up always seeing something, particularly something benign like dogs or cats, it would never occur to you that they
weren't real. They'd just blend in with everything else and you'd never
know the difference between reality and hallucination until you got
old enough to realize other people weren't seeing what you were.

I look up at the lights again, trying to imagine what she's seeing,
but I can't do it. I turn back to her. "What did you do today? Did you
make anything in art therapy?"

"I went to Calilini," Jani answers, still staring at the lights above.

"When did you go?"

"Earlier today."

"Jani, you've been on the unit all day. You never left."

"Yes, I did," she answers languidly, as if I am a fading voice in a
dream.

"Then how come no one saw you?"

"I go at night."

I know this isn't true. Jani sleeps at night because of the medication. I know she is watched and the unit is locked. But I also know
that none of this means anything to Jani.

"You mean you go there in your head?"

"No, I actually go."

"How do you get out?"

"Dogs come and get me. Great Danes."

"Great Danes are pretty big dogs, Jani. Too big to not be seen."

"They take me to visit my friends in Calilini. I ride on their back."

I lie down next to her again, my face inches from hers. "The next time they come, can you call me? I want to go to Calilini, too."

"You can't."

"Why can't I go, too? I want to see Calilini."

"You're too big to ride the Great Danes, and that's the only way to get there."

I roll over and sit up, upset. I can't see what she sees, but I want her to guide me. Sadly, I realize she now equates me with this world. *I don't want to be part of this world, Jani. I want to go with you.*

"Jani," I ask, pushing down my emotions again. I need information. "What's the temperature in Calilini right now?"

Over the past few weeks, I have learned that the temperature in Calilini seems to correlate to her level of psychosis. When it is high, above 140 degrees, it means she's getting more psychotic. A few weeks ago, when they raised her Thorazine level to 300mg daily, it started dropping: first to 120, then 110, then 100. It got as low as 85 degrees. Her "autistic-like" hand wringing even stopped, but then she went into dystonia again and they had to pull back on the dosage. Since then, the temperature has been creeping up again.

"One hundred and eighty," Jani answers.

Almost boiling point.

CHAPTER THIRTY-FOUR

Late April 2009

This semester I am teaching two classes, the minimum required to keep my health insurance benefits. I'm at my desk when yet another student enters late. I look up at the clock. It's 4:45 P.M. Class started twenty minutes ago, but I still haven't done anything. I've just been sitting at the desk.

He takes a seat in the front row just a few feet from me.

"Where were you?" I ask, my voice deep and dangerous.

He takes out his phone and texts in front of me.

"Huh? Oh, sorry." He looks up at me. "I was at the gym and then I had to take a shower." He returns to texting.

I'm silent for a moment. "When I was a student," I finally say, "I at least had enough respect for my professors to lie when I was late."

This student looks up at me, a smile on his face because he thinks I'm joking. I glare at him. *My daughter has schizophrenia. It's getting worse and nobody seems to be able to stop it. Pieces of my daughter's mind are eroding like chunks ripped away from the sandy bank of a rain-swollen river.*

"If you can't make it to a class on time," I look him straight in the eye, "why should anyone believe you'll make it to a job on time? Do you really think that when you get that nice little business administration degree your life is going to change? It won't. You know why?"

He doesn't answer, his cell phone hanging limply in his hands, his text forgotten.

"Because," I continue, my voice meaner, "when you graduate from this college, it will be alongside millions of other students with the same degree. This isn't Harvard. There's nothing special about you that'll make you stand out from the millions of other stupid punks with the same degree. Any idiot can get a college degree."

My eyes scan across the room. "That goes for all of you. What high school guidance counselors tell you about college is bullshit. A college degree doesn't fundamentally change who you are. If you were a loser before college, you'll be a loser after it . . . just a loser with a worthless piece of paper that gives you a false sense of hope that your life is going to amount to something, but you know where you will end up working after college, assuming you can even find a job? Selling insurance, or telemarketing."

In the back of my mind I'm vaguely aware that I am losing it, but I don't care anymore. I lean forward over the podium, staring into their stunned faces.

"The truth is you are going to end up working in a cubicle for the rest of your life, until you die. If any of you had brains in your head, I might actually believe you could fight your way up, but look at you! Half of you can't even make it to an *afternoon* class on time. You're nothing but a number. Enjoy your cubicle." I start packing up my briefcase.

"Are you leaving?" a female student asks nervously.

I swing my bag over my shoulder. "I'm done wasting my time with all of you. I have better things to do." And I walk out.

I'M SITTING IN my car parked in the faculty lot, trying to light a cigarette, but my hands are shaking so badly that the flame on the lighter keeps going out. As I was leaving, I caught a glimpse of the stunned looks on my students' faces. In four years of teaching, I've never lost my cool in front of a class. I was teaching when Jani went into Alhambra and when I got accused of sexual molestation, but I didn't lose my cool. I was teaching when Jani's diagnosis officially became schizophrenia, and I didn't lose my cool. For a year and a half I've gone through this nightmare and never lost my cool . . . until today.

I finally manage to light my cigarette and take a long drag. I've been living two separate lives, one as Jani's father and the other as Professor Schofield, but I can't do it anymore. I'm the father of a child who is losing her mind to a disease nobody can stop. I can't fake being the other guy anymore.

I call Susan and tell her what happened.

"Just come home," she gently suggests. "Come home and we'll be together."

I shake my head vehemently. "It's my night to visit Jani. I have to take her the food she requested."

"I've already called the unit," Susan replies. "She's asleep."

I'm not surprised. She's already asleep most nights by the time I arrive for visiting hours. The medications knock her out early.

"It was a rough day, but she is fine now. She is sleeping peacefully. Just come home. Please." She's begging me to come home, but it doesn't sound like the old days, when she'd been out with Jani all day and she would call me constantly, asking me when I was coming home from work. It's different now. Jani is not there. I don't need to race back to take care of her.

I realize Susan is begging me to come home because of me. I'm going over the edge and she is trying to pull me back.

"No," I tell her. "I need to go see Jani, even if she is asleep. I need to do it for me and make sure she's okay." My voice breaks and I clear my throat. "I will call you when I'm on my way home." I hang up.

A NURSE IS sitting outside Jani's room, and I already know something is wrong. The only reason a nurse would be there is if Jani got assigned a "one-to-one," meaning she was a danger to herself or others. I have never seen this nurse before. She doesn't have a UCLA ID. Must be a temp.

"She's asleep," she tells me in a heavy West African accent.

"She'll wake up for the food," I reply and go into the dark room, where I see the outline of Jani in her bed.

I step forward and hear the sound of paper scuffling under my feet. I reach down and pull the paper from my shoe. I turn on the light and see that it's a page torn from a Dora the Explorer book, a Ready-to-Read book. Jani has known how to read since she was two. We bought these books for her back then and kept them for Bodhi since she'd outgrown them, but these are the books she asks us to bring now. I don't know why. I try to bring her educational books, but she doesn't want those. She wants these simple books where one sentence takes up the entire page. Maybe they comfort her, reminding her of a simpler time, her way of trying to go back.

I look up and see the room is strewn with shreds of paper. I put the food on her desk and start picking them up.

Gillian, the charge nurse whom we've come to know, enters the room and sees me picking up the mess.

"She ripped up all her books," she tells me, sadness in her voice. "She tried to destroy all of her stuff. We had to lock everything away."

I pick up a crumpled piece of paper and my legs give way. I sit down hard on the floor, staring at the piece of paper. It's a page from one of her Winnie-the-Pooh books, the original Winnie-the-Pooh chapter books, the page faded into a light yellow. They were nearly sixty years old, given to my father in 1953 for his fifth birthday. When I was a kid, he gave them to me. When Jani was old enough, I passed them on to her. I'm numb. She destroyed books that have been in my family for three generations.

"I'll have someone come in to clean up the mess," Gillian says.

"No," I answer. "It's okay. I got it."

"You sure?" Gillian asks. I look at her and realize she, too, is worried about me.

"Yep," I say, picking up some of the pieces.

"You okay?" Gillian asks me.

"Fine," I answer automatically.

She hesitates. "Okay. Call me if you need anything."

"Wait."

Gillian turns back.

"Did she get her last dose of meds?"

Gillian hesitates. "No," she finally answers. "She fell asleep before she could take them. If she wakes up, let me know so I can give her her meds."

She leaves and I begin to pick up more torn pages. I look down at the Winnie-the-Pooh pages for a moment, then push the whole lot down in the trash. I don't want her to wake up and be confronted with what she did. When she wakes up, I want to spend happy times with her.

I turn to Jani, passed out on the bed, still in her clothes. "Jani!" I call loudly. "Daddy's here!"

Jani's eyes open.

I feel a sense of relief that I am able to wake her without too much effort. "Hey, sweetie!" I say, sitting on the edge of her bed.

She sits up, stringy hair falling about her face. She looks around like she just woke up from a dream and is trying to remember where she is.

"I brought you Burger King like you asked." I brush the hair out of her face.

She turns to me, staring for a second.

"Who are you?" she asks.

My blood freezes in my veins. No, I think to myself, she must be joking. We've always been silly with each other.

"Who am I?" I repeat, smiling, waiting for her to grin and rub her hands, acknowledging the joke.

But the grin and the excited hand rubbing don't come. She just keeps staring at me as if she's never seen me before in her life.

The smile on my face fades as the truth sinks in. My worst nightmare has come to pass: She doesn't recognize me anymore.

"I'm your daddy," I tell her, in an amazingly level voice.

"Oh," she answers and looks around the room.

"I brought food for you."

"I'm not hungry." .

She puts her head back down on the pillow.

I reach forward and pull her into my arms. I don't want her to go back to sleep. I don't want to let her go.

"Do you want to watch TV?"

"I'm tired," she answers, hanging in my arms.

"Come on. Watch TV with me. *Survivorman* might be on." I try to get her to reconnect with her past. We used to watch *Survivorman* together.

"I just want to sleep." She pulls free of me and sags back onto the bed.

In the six years of her life, I have never known Jani to "just want to sleep."

"Jani," I ask. "What's the temperature in Calilini?"

"Two hundred," she mumbles.

Twelve degrees to go.

I CALL SUSAN on my way home.

"How was she?" Susan asks when she picks up the phone. "She must have been awake, because you were there a long time. I've been waiting for you to call."

"She didn't know who I was."

Silence for a moment, just windblast outside my window, and taillights from cars I barely see driving ahead in the distance.

"What do you mean she didn't know who you were?" Susan finally asks.

"She was asleep when I got there. When I woke her up . . . she . . . she asked me who I was."

Silence.

"At first I thought she was joking, playing a game with me, but she wasn't. She just stared at me. She really had no idea who I was."

I hear Susan sniffle on the other end. She's crying.

"Do you have Bodhi?"

"He's sleeping in my arms."

"Good." *That's where I want him. Hold him, Susan, and never let him go.*

"He's such a sweet boy," Susan says, her voice filled with agony.

"Yes, he is. I'm glad you have him."

"You know, I've been thinking . . . ," Susan begins.

"Yeah?"

"What if the reason Jani wanted a sibling wasn't for her, but for us?"

I can't speak.

"Maybe she knew. She knew she was going and we couldn't live without her. She wanted us to have Bodhi because she wanted to give us something to keep going."

This is excruciating. Everything outside the windshield begins to blur as tears come. But it is not hard to believe Susan is right. We have said for years that we could not go on if something happened to Jani.

"I remember," Susan says, "she once told me, 'I feel like I'm living on the border between your world and my world.'"

I am thinking of a dream Susan had that she told me about recently. In it, she was taking Bodhi to his first day of kindergarten at the same elementary school in San Mateo, south of San Francisco, that she went to as a kid. Neither Jani nor I was in the dream. I asked Susan where we were. She looked confused for a moment. "I don't know," she said. "You weren't there."

"What do you want to do?" Susan asks me now.

"I want to bring her home."

"I understand. Bring her home. We'll find a way to deal with it. We'll make it."

But Susan doesn't understand.

"I can't bring her home while Bodhi is still there. She's still a danger to him." I suck my breath in. I know Susan isn't going to like this. "I want you to take him and go to your parents in San Mateo."

"No!" Susan cries, the tears breaking free again.

"He's suffered enough. He deserves a life."

"But I want to be here for her! She's my daughter, too!"

"I understand that, and you've done a great job. There's no one else I'd rather have gone through this with. We kept her alive for six years. All the people who told us that we shouldn't let her dominate our lives were wrong."

"She always had it," Susan says. "I remember when she was a

baby, her looking around, watching something we couldn't see, but together, we kept it at bay by taking her out all the time."

"Yes, we did, but we can't anymore. It is too strong. Bodhi needs his mommy. He needs you more than he needs me." My mind drifts back to when I took off my wedding ring for the MRI, how soldiers remove all personal effects before going into a battle they don't know they'll come back from.

"That's not true! He needs his daddy!" Susan cries.

"He's still young enough that he won't remember me. Or Jani. He'll grow up and he'll be fine. It's better for him to lose me now than later, when he's old enough to remember."

"I don't want him to lose you at all!"

"I know that. I don't want to lose him. I want to see my son grow up. I've never really gotten the chance to know him. I thought Jani would be with me, and together she and I would teach him all the things I taught her."

"I don't want to lose my daughter."

"If Bodhi is not here, I can bring her home. I will take care of her. And whatever happens, happens."

"And what then?"

"Remember that dream you had? The one where you were taking Bodhi to his first day of school in San Mateo? Jani and I weren't there."

"It was a dream!" Susan argues. "I had it years before Bodhi was even born. Besides, you and Jani could have been somewhere else."

"Maybe it wasn't," I answer. "Maybe it was a vision of the future."

"I can't believe this is happening!" Susan cries. She's been saying this ever since Alhambra. It doesn't change anything.

"Jani and I will come up to visit if we can, and you can come down to visit." I'm lying. I am not sure we will ever make it to that point. If Jani leaves our world completely, I don't see how I can go on.

I know there is still Bodhi and I know Bodhi would still need me, but without Jani nothing else matters to me. Maybe it's weakness. Maybe it's selfishness.

"No," Susan replies, her voice suddenly strong.

"It's the only way," I repeat.

"It's not the only way," she fires back. "It can't be the only way. There has to be another."

"There isn't," I say angrily, hanging up.

TWENTY MINUTES LATER, I'm still driving, taking the long way home, when my cell phone rings. I can see it is Susan. I don't want to keep rehashing this. I've made my decision.

"Yes?" I answer.

"I just got an idea." She's not crying. She sounds excited. "I was praying to God for an answer and it came to me. It came from God. I know it."

I sigh. "What?"

"The only reason she can't come home is because of Bodhi, right?"

"Yes," I reply.

"So what if we get two apartments?"

"I can't afford two apartments."

"No, I mean, what if we trade in this apartment for two smaller apartments, two one-bedrooms. One would be Bodhi's apartment and one would be Jani's. You and I could trade off, alternating nights. One night you stay with Jani and I stay with Bodhi, and the next night we switch. What do you think? Brilliant, huh?"

I am stunned into silence.

"We could keep the kids separated," she goes on, "but still stay together as a family. It's from God, I'm telling you. Tomorrow I'm going to go talk to the leasing office and see if there are any one-bedrooms available."

For the first time in a long time, something stirs within me. It takes me a few seconds to realize it is hope. I have to be crazy to have hope now.

"What do you think?" Susan asks me.

"Honestly, I think it's crazy."

"So do I. Which is why I think it might work."

261

CHAPTER THIRTY-FIVE

May 15, 2009

I t's moving day. I stand in the middle of our two-bedroom apartment with the moving men, pointing at each piece of furniture.

"The kitchen table goes to Bodhi's apartment," I tell them. "The couch goes to Jani's apartment."

We are dividing up our possessions, splitting our home.

Susan's family thinks what we're doing is insane, but Jani has forced Susan and me to live apart since she was a baby. This is just a more extreme version of that separation.

All of the cooking supplies are going to Bodhi's apartment, for safety reasons. There will be no glass or ceramics in Jani's apartment, nothing she can use to hurt herself. Nothing she can pick up and throw.

The goal with Jani's apartment is to create a minature version of the UCLA child psych unit. We're no longer trying to re-integrate Jani into our lives, but are instead altering our existence to fit what works for her. At UCLA, there is a dry-erase board in each room that tells the child "Good Morning" along with his or her assigned staff, so I hang up a dry-erase board that lists which parent is Jani's "staff" for the day. In the day room at UCLA, another dry-erase board lists planned activities from the time the kids get up until they go to bed. I hang up a similar board in Jani's living room, listing her daily schedule, which includes "recreational therapy" and "occupational therapy" just like in the hospital. Recreational therapy will be going outside and playing. For occupational/art therapy I go to Michaels Crafts and load up on arts and crafts projects, which fill the cupboards of Jani's kitchen so her apartment is entirely set up for therapeutic purposes.

On her schedule board I write *Dinner (Go to Bodhi's)* in the 5 P.M. slot. We'll eat meals at exactly the same time Jani eats at UCLA. I worry about taking her over to Bodhi's, even for just an hour, but Susan and I feel it is important to be together, to remind ourselves that we're still a family. Splitting up is, ironically, the only way to keep our family together. This way Bodhi can have his space, free to explore his world without fear of what Jani might do, and Jani doesn't have to worry about hurting Bodhi. And most importantly, Susan and I no longer have to live in fear every second.

I rub my hands over the walls of Jani's old bedroom, over the words she wrote during her time-outs. I tried washing them off, scrubbing for hours, but could never completely erase them. My hand pauses over the outline of *400*, scrawled in giant numbers above where her bed used to be. *I'm sorry, Jani,* I think to myself. *I didn't know.*

I walk out of her bedroom and leave the keys on the mantel, glad to be leaving this apartment. I never want to see those walls again.

June 1, 2009

Today is discharge day. Jani has been in UCLA for more than four months, making her the longest continuous resident on the child and adolescent psychiatric unit in decades. Dr. Kim and UCLA knew we needed time to get into the two separate apartments, so they fought off Blue Shield until we completed the move.

"I think it is great idea," Dr. Kim said when we told her our plan. "It's really thinking outside of the box."

I look down the discharge sheet that Dr. Kim has handed me to sign and see *Discharge Diagnosis*. Next to it, handwritten, is the word *Schizophrenia*. The word stares me in the face. It's the first time I've seen it written on a medical report that has to do with Jani. My six-year-old daughter is now officially labeled with the most severe mental illness in the world.

Below the discharge diagnosis is *Expected Course of Recovery*, with three boxes that can be checked: *good, fair,* and *poor prognosis*. Kim hasn't checked a box yet. She sees me looking at it.

"Sorry. Forgot that one," she says, removing a pen from her pocket. She checks *fair*.

Fair. Not quite good, but not quite poor, either. Fair is right down the middle. Fair is a C in college. I'm not sure whether she really believes that or if she just wants to give us hope. It doesn't matter, though. It wouldn't change what we're doing.

I sign my name at the bottom of the page. Dr. Kim hands me my copies and looks up. "I just want to say that I have really enjoyed working with all of you these past few months. Jani is a very special, very intelligent little girl."

"What do you think will happen to her?" I ask Dr. Kim.

Kim sighs. "I think . . . I wouldn't let go of hope."

I smile. "You're a doctor. You have to say that."

"I'm not saying it as a doctor. I'm saying it as someone who has come to care deeply about Jani and your family. I have hope she will make it."

I offer my hand and she shakes it. Her time as a fellow is over, and she is now rotating off of the unit. Chances are I will never see her again. Despite myself, I reach out and embrace her.

"Thank you," I say.

She hugs me back, breaking the rule that says doctors are supposed to maintain a certain distance.

"For what? Jani has gotten better because she has worked very hard."

"Thank you for having faith in her," I answer.

"I have a lot of faith in her," she tells me as we break off the hug. "I also have a lot of faith in you and Susan."

I nod, unable to meet her eyes. As hard as I try, I cannot find faith of my own. Jani is better, but "better" is a relative term. Dr. Kim speaks of Jani's "baseline of psychosis," meaning the level of psychosis that is "normal" for her. Now we have to see how well, or even if, she can function at all outside of the structured and secure environment of the hospital.

It is time to go. I'm carrying two suitcases plus three full-sized plastic bags that contain everything we've brought, along with all the art therapy projects Jani's made in the last four months.

"You ready to go, Jani?"

Jani hugs each of the nurses and Dr. Kim. A few of them are tearing up. None of them has worked with a child as long as they have all worked with Jani. Watching her say good-bye, it feels like they are more her family now than we are.

Done with her good-byes, she turns to me, holding Hero.

"You ready to see your new apartment?" I ask.

She rubs her hands together, excitedly. "Can 24 Hours come, too?"

I pause, remembering what Dr. Kim told me in our last family session. *In all likelihood, the hallucinations will never completely go away.*

"Sure," I reluctantly reply.

Jani turns back to the empty corridor. "Come on, 24 Hours! Let's go!"

WE FINISH OUR dinner.

"Who is my staff tonight?" Jani asks. "Mommy or Daddy?"

I'm cleaning the dishes. "Who do you want?"

"Mommy," Jani answers.

"Okay." Susan smiles.

I don't mind. Jani needs to get used to spending time with Susan again, and I've never spent a night alone with Bodhi.

Jani comes over to Susan. "Can we go now?"

"Sure," Susan replies, gathering her clothes for tomorrow. Most of her clothes are here, while most of mine are in Jani's apartment. I'm not sure why I told the movers to put the boxes with my clothes in Jani's apartment. Maybe I don't really want to alternate nights.

I hug Jani good-bye. "I'll see you tomorrow, okay?"

"Okay," she answers, more relaxed than I've seen her since Bodhi was born. She likes this arrangement. When I asked her why on the drive home from the hospital, she said, "So Bodhi won't get into my stuff and I won't hit him."

I think having her own place, away from Bodhi, has taken an immense amount of stress off her. She doesn't have to fight with her mind every minute to not hurt Bodhi.

I kiss her on top of her head. She opens the door.

"Come on," she calls to Susan.

"Coming," Susan replies.

We lean toward each other and quickly kiss, then she's out the door after Jani. I can't remember the last time we kissed. With a shock I realize it was the night before Bodhi was born. We haven't kissed in almost two years.

Bodhi starts to cry, realizing Susan is gone. I go over to him and pick him up in my arms. "It's okay, little guy, Daddy's here. You'll see Mommy tomorrow."

I stand in the middle of his apartment, holding him, trying to console him. His mother is gone for the first time ever.

I go to the window, push aside the blinds, and look out, seeing Susan and Jani crossing the parking lot. I watch them until they disappear into Jani's apartment.

Sunday, June 7, 2009

I have to take Honey out. It's been so long since she's run freely. I tell Susan over the phone that we should all go as a family up to the local high school.

"Can't you just take Honey for a walk around the complex?" Susan asks me. "I can watch both kids for ten minutes."

"Honey needs longer than ten minutes. She needs to run and roam freely."

"I know," Susan admits. "But let's wait until Dave and Cameron get here. Besides, it's hot and Jani burns easily on the Thorazine." The only thing keeping Jani in our world at all is 200mg of Thorazine. Unfortunately, one of its side effects is extreme photosensitivity.

"I can put lots of sunblock on," I reply.

"Why won't you just take Honey for a walk and come back? We can always go later when they're here."

I suddenly get angry. "Because I want to have a normal day together as a family. Can't we just have that for once? I'm not even asking for time alone. I just want one day as a family."

"I think we're taking a risk," Susan warns.

"It'll be fine. I'll bring toys, food, and water. We can have a picnic up there."

. . .

IT'S HOTTER THAN I had expected, so I set up the toys in the shade by the tennis courts. I hope to keep Jani engaged for a few hours, playing with me. Just like old times.

"Jani, let's scooter," I call to her, seeing her scratching the top of her head roughly.

"My head is itchy," she whines.

"It's the Thorazine," Susan says, sitting with Bodhi in the shade.

I feel anger building up inside of me. "It's not the Thorazine," I shoot back. "We just got here. She's got sunblock on and she's in the frickin' shade. It's a tactile hallucination." Jani's hallucinations are not limited to sights and sounds. All five of her senses experience hallucinations.

"It's too hot," Jani complains.

"It's not that hot," I answer her. "It's still in the eighties."

"I'm hot," Susan says, "so I can imagine she is."

"You're not helping!" I glare at her.

"I want to go," Jani announces, still tearing at her scalp.

"No. Honey hasn't had any time to run yet."

"I think we should go," Susan says. "This was a bad idea."

I can feel myself losing control of my emotions. I am getting angry as I sense my "family day" falling to pieces.

"I just wanted us to have fun as a family. Is that such a bad idea? At least I'm trying, which is more than I can say for you."

"Did you take your Lexapro this morning?" Susan asks.

"It's in Bodhi's apartment," I answer.

"You need your medication," Susan says sternly.

"It was in Bodhi's apartment!"

"You need to take it so you don't get like this," Susan says.

"No, you need to back me up so I don't get like this," I retort. "Jani, get back here now."

Jani, already at the car, reluctantly comes back.

"Okay, do you want to play dog ball?" I ask her, which is where we throw a tennis ball to Honey.

Instead, Jani gets on Bodhi's toddler train and pushes herself along. She looks ridiculous. I remember reading about schizophrenia eating away the gray matter of the brain. She was a genius and now she's riding a toddler's toy.

Dave and Cameron pull into the parking lot and Cameron leaps out, running up to Honey, who's already barking at him.

He recoils.

"Honey!" I yell at her, then to Cameron, "Don't be afraid! Dogs pick up on fear!"

Honey jumps and nips at Cameron, and he flinches away.

"Cameron, are you okay?!" Susan gets up with Bodhi in her arms and rushes to him as I grab Honey.

"He's okay." Dave's walking faster than normal, sweating in the heat. "The kid's done far worse to me."

"I'm hot!" Jani screams, getting off Bodhi's train. She returns to scratching her scalp.

"You want me to fix it?" I ask.

She nods. I take a bottle of water and slowly pour some over her head to cool her off.

"Feel better?" I ask.

Jani nods. Then she looks down and sees that water has spilled onto her shirt. Her eyes open wide and she screams.

"I'm wet!" She tugs her shirt off.

"Jani, what are you doing?"

"I have to get new clothes!" she cries.

"It's just water. It's a hot day. It will keep you cool."

But Jani is stripping off her clothes.

"I have to take her home," I say.

"We need to all go," Susan says.

I look back at Jani, pulling off everything right in front of Cameron.

"Jani! Stop that!"

"I'm wet!" she cries again.

"Fine, we'll go home and get you new clothes."

"We should all go."

"No, I'm not taking Bodhi back with Honey. Honey will step on him and he'll cry, then Jani will fly into a rage. Just stay here and we'll be back." We all came up together and we're still going to have a picnic. I refuse to give up on my dream of a "normal" day.

I get Honey into the car. "Jani! Let's go." My voice is angry. I'm angry. *All I want is for us to have some fun as a family, but either the schizophrenia or the drug to treat it keeps getting in the way. Is this how it's going to be for the rest of our lives?*

"And please take your Lexapro!" Susan begs.

Jani cries that she's burning.

"You were just complaining about being wet!" I yell. "If you don't want to burn, put your clothes back on."

Jani does, crying like I'm abusing her. This is not what I wanted. I wanted a fun day for Jani to look back on, to replace the fun days with me she no longer remembers.

"It's still wet," Jani cries.

"Then get in the damn car!"

"You're scaring her," Susan calls to me. "Maybe I should take her. Jani, do you want to go with Mommy?"

"We'll be fine," I yell. But I'm not fine. I haven't felt fine in years.

I floor the car out of the parking lot and into the street. The speedometer hits fifty, sixty, then seventy. I look over at Jani and realize she isn't wearing her seat belt. She always fights me on that, too. I should slow down. I should buckle her up. But I don't. Instead, I reach down and release the catch on my own seat belt. I look over at the streetlamps flying past. One flick of my wrist and we'd plow right into one. I'd go through the windshield and everything would be over. I want it to be over.

For two years I have hovered on the edge. Now I am going over it. The fundamental requirement for survival is faith and I don't have it. I don't know if Jani will get better or worse. I don't know anything.

Jani is screaming, but not from my driving. She is screaming about her phantom sunburn.

I think about my Lexapro. Normally I'm supposed to take two pills. But I just got a refill. There are sixty pills in the bottle, each pill 20mg.

Jani is ripping at the top of her skull with her fingers.

"Jani, stop that! You're gonna make yourself bleed!"

"But it's so itchy!"

I think about the Lexapro again. Twelve hundred milligrams total. It's just an antidepressant. Can you overdose on an antidepressant? Maybe if I really want to end it, I should swallow a bottle of one of Jani's medications. They do nothing for her, but they would probably kill me.

Twelve hundred milligrams. Would that be enough to initiate organ shutdown? Would it stop my heart?

I'm driving thirty miles over the speed limit, hoping to hear a siren behind me. I want to be arrested. I'm tired of being "strong." I never was "strong." I can't fix what she has. I can't even make her life better.

My cell rings. I know it's Susan without having to look at it. She is calling, probably worried, as she should be, but I don't answer. If I answer, she'll try to talk me down, and I don't want to be talked down.

I pull into our parking space, get out, and go around to the other side of the car. I wrench open the back passenger door. "Honey, get out!" Honey doesn't move. She's scared and shaking. "Dammit, Honey!" I grab her leash and yank with all my strength. Honey falls out onto the pavement and I drag her as she struggles to regain her feet.

Jani jumps out, her face worried. "Don't hurt Honey!" she cries.

"What do you care? You hurt Honey all the time." It's strange to be aware of your own mental and emotional breakdown. I know I should stop. But I don't. I want to lash out and hurt someone, anyone, like I've been hurting for so long.

I head for the stairs of the building Bodhi's apartment is in. I realize Jani is not following. I look down and see her at the bottom of the stairwell, staring up at me.

"Jani, get up here!" I yell down at her.

"I'll stay here."

"Jani, get up here now!" I roar so loud my voice goes hoarse.

Jani reluctantly starts climbing the stairs after me.

We get into Bodhi's apartment. I let go of Honey. It's cool and dark inside the apartment. I go to the bathroom, retrieve a washcloth, and run it under cold water, then squeeze it out and tell Jani to lie down on the bed. I lay it across her face.

"How's that? Feel better?" I ask, my voice now completely calm.

"Yes."

"Okay." She's been taken care of. I turn from her, go into the kitchen, and pour a cup of water. Then I open the medicine cabinet, seeing all the pill bottles, most of them full from medications prescribed for Jani that were tried and abandoned.

There is my Lexapro. I open the bottle and toss back my head, fill my mouth with tablets, so many that I feel like I'm going to choke. I lift the cup of water to my lips and drink, my mouth so full that water spills out the sides of my lips and runs down my face.

Reason tries to regain control of me. *What are you doing?!* I don't know. I don't care. I don't want to think. *You could still spit them out,* the voice in my head tells me. I ignore it and swallow. It takes several gulps to get the all the pills down. I feel a sharp pain in my throat as the muscles fight to get the solid block of tablets down. *I can still spit out what is left.* I take another swig of water, then another, continuing to swallow.

Finally, my mouth is empty. I look down at the bottle, still half-full. Dammit. I'm going to have to do this again. I put the bottle to my lips and toss back my head.

"Daddy?" I hear softly behind me.

I turn to Jani, the half-empty bottle of Lexapro still in my hand.

"I found a new pair of pants." I look down and see her holding them out to me. "Can you help me get dressed?"

I drop the bottle of pills and they scatter across the floor in all directions. A sob comes out of my mouth like vomit.

My body buckles under the weight of six years of emotional repression. My feet slide down the kitchen cabinet, my shirt ripping as it catches on the metal handle of a drawer.

The dam has broken. I wail uncontrollably, tears streaming down my face.

"Daddy?" Jani stands in front of me, scared. She takes a step closer and reaches out her hand and pats the top of my head. "It'll be okay, Daddy."

No, it won't, Jani. It will never be okay again. You have something I can't save you from.

"I'm feeling better now," she says.

I can't speak. All I can do is look up at her. Right now she seems so normal. But she isn't. And she never will be.

"Why are you crying, Daddy?"

I'm crying for you . . . for me . . . for Susan and Bodhi. I'm crying for everything we lost and everything we will never have.

.   .   .

THE CLOCK IS ticking now. I don't know how many pills I've swallowed. Am I dying? I have no idea what will happen to me, but I know I don't want Jani to see it. I have to get her back to Susan.

I pull myself to my feet. "Come on."

"Where are we going?"

"I need to get you back to Mommy."

We are driving up Valencia Boulevard when I spot Dave's truck coming in the opposite direction. I pull a U-turn and follow them back into our apartment complex. Dave is parking his truck in our space.

Susan walks toward my car with Bodhi in her arms. I stop the car in the middle of the parking lot, right between Jani's apartment and Bodhi's apartment.

"Get out and go to Mommy," I tell Jani.

"Where are you going?" she asks, looking at me, worried.

I don't immediately know what to say. "I need some time."

Jani gets out and runs over to Susan, leaving the car door open. I reach over and pull it closed. Out the windshield I see Susan talking to Jani.

Susan comes over, holding Bodhi in her arms. I lower the window.

"I asked Jani if you hurt Honey," she says, looking disturbed. "She said you yelled but you didn't."

But I did. Jani saw me. She doesn't remember. It doesn't matter what I do anymore. Jani won't remember.

"I yanked her out of the car pretty hard," I confess. I could have lied. But I don't want to. I know hurting Honey will make Susan angry, and I want her to be angry. It will make it easier to leave.

Susan's face screws up in fear.

"Jani or Honey?"

"Honey."

"Why?" Her voice is breaking. "Why did you do that? She's a defenseless animal." She looks at me like I'm a monster.

"I overdosed on my Lexapro," I softly say.

Susan just stares at me.

"Why would you do that?" she finally manages to say.

I realize I don't have an answer. "I don't know. I just did."

She shakes her head sadly. "You just made our lives even harder."

"I just tried to kill myself and that is all you can say?"

"What do you want me to say?" she replies. "Am I upset? Yes, but I have to take care of Jani and Bodhi."

And that is what it comes down to, I realize. It's not that we don't love each other. We can't. There is no energy to muster love after Jani. What was I expecting? Her to take me in her arms and beg for me to live? She can't do that. She has to take care of Bodhi. And Jani.

"You need to go to the hospital."

"No. I'm going to drive into the desert and let the pills do their thing."

Susan looks away again. For the first time in my life, I see what love and hate look like in the same face. That's it. That is what we've both felt ever since Jani was born, love and hate at the same time.

Bodhi starts to cry.

"I can't deal with this now," Susan says and turns away, heading for Jani.

I drive away.

I drive up Valencia Boulevard and turn right on Westridge Parkway. I wonder if Susan will call the police. I have no idea. I'm going to take this road until it dead-ends at the top of a canyon and then leave the car. I have to leave the car so they don't find me. I will hike down into the canyon as far as I can go. I hiked down there once before, with Jani. We went farther than I expected, until Jani stopped and wanted to go back. I stood there for a minute, knowing she would go back without me, so I ran after her. I've been chasing after her her whole life.

I take my foot off the gas and the car gradually eases to a stop in the middle of the road.

What will they do when I'm gone? What will Susan do? What will Jani do? What will Bodhi do?

The car continues idling in the middle of the road.

I'm abandoning them to find their own way without me just because I can't deal with the fact that I don't know what to do.

I sigh.

I can't do this. I have to go back.

I step on the gas again and spin the wheel, turning the car around.

SUSAN IS SITTING on the stairwell, talking on the phone, when I walk up.

"He just came back," she says into the phone.

I sit down next to her.

"Where's Jani and Bo . . . Bodhi?" I slur, as the pills start taking their effect.

"Dave took them to the pool. They're fine."

"Can we . . . can we talk?"

"I'll call you back," she says into the phone. "Yes, he's here now. I don't know if he needs to go to the hospital."

She looks up at me. "Do you need to go to the hospital?"

"I can't." I'm very tired now. "If I go . . . if I go . . . tif igo . . ." Shit. I can't get a sentence out.

"He's slurring his speech," Susan says into the phone. "Tracy says you need to go to the hospital so they can pump your stomach."

I have to focus on my words. "If I go to the hospital, they'll put me on a . . . on a three-day hold. . . . because I attempted suicide. I will . . . be there at least three days, maybe longer. What . . . will you do? You . . . will be alone with the . . . kids."

"I will be alone with the kids anyway if you die." She is not scared. She is angry. Angry at me. I understand.

"I have to . . . try and walk it off."

"Is that possible?"

I smile. Or at least I think I smile. I can't feel my face. "I hope so."

"But you need to be with Bodhi tonight!"

"I don't . . . I don't think I should. . . . I think I should be with Jani tonight. Bodhi wakes up and I might not wake up. I don't want him to wake up screaming for a bottle and I can't respond. Jani sleeps through the . . . night now." I pause, struck by the fact that that used to be my biggest concern. "I have to stay up as long as I can . . . to give the Lexapro time to drain out of my system."

I want to fall over, but I fight it.

Of course, what if Jani wakes up tomorrow morning to find me cold and lifeless next to her? Which is better? Which child would I rather find me dead?

Susan hangs up the phone. "I think you need to go to the hospital."

"I'll . . . be okay."

"Why did you do this?" she asks me. "Why now? After everything we've been through, and now things are getting better."

I turn to her. "Because they're not getting better."

She looks perplexed. "What do you mean, 'they're not getting better'? They're better than they were. Jani is better than she was. She's not as violent anymore."

"Only because she is taking enough Thorazine to put a horse in a coma. She's not really any better. Every drug she has ever been on either hasn't worked at all or stopped working after a period of time. What will we do when the Thorazine stops working?"

Susan looks away. "We'll deal with that if and when it happens."

"You don't get it," I reply angrily. "Look at everything we've done just to get her to this point."

"I am. And it's working."

"But we won't live forever."

She turns back to me. "So why are you trying to speed that up?"

I open my mouth to reply, but then it finally sinks in.

Why are you trying to speed that up?

Why do I want to die?

Because I'm afraid of watching Jani slowly die in front of my eyes while I am powerless to stop it. Deep down, I realize I've been planning this ever since I asked Dr. Kim Jani's prognosis. *Fifty-fifty.* Schizophrenics statistically have a shorter life span than the rest of the population. On that day the diagnosis became official, for the first time since Jani was born, it occurred to me that she might die before me.

I can't bear that.

"Because I don't want to outlive my daughter," I answer. "I don't want her to die."

Susan looks at me. "But everyone faces that possibility. Any of us could get hit by a bus tomorrow. We're just more aware of it."

"I don't want to be aware."

Susan puts her arm around me. "I can't promise you she will always be okay."

"I wish you could."

"You have to have faith. This is what faith is all about. We have to do whatever we can to make her as happy as possible for as long as we have."

"I can't make her happy."

"Yes, you can. You always have."

"Not anymore. I don't know how to reach her anymore."

"It will get better. I don't know how I know, but I just do. I have a gut feeling. We just have to hang on."

I look at her. I don't believe her.

"I've never had blind faith in anything," I answer.

"But this is what faith truly is. I believe in God and I believe we were given Jani for a reason. You know as well as I do that she's always been special. This is just our challenge. Other people have their challenges, too. They have kids who are blind, deaf, or in wheelchairs. Jani can still run and play. She's lucky."

. . .

"I'M SORRY . . . I'M sorry, Jani. I can't . . . I can't read tonight."

I am lying in bed next to Jani, fighting the desire to close my eyes. I must stay up. The longer I stay awake, the better the chance I'll wake up tomorrow morning.

"Mommy will read to me tomorrow."

"I'm . . . sorry. We can . . . we can watch TV? *SpongeBob*?"

Jani pulls up her blankets.

"I'm tired." I look over at her, sensing she knows what I've done.

I tuck Hero Bear into her arms and she snuggles into him.

"Jani?"

"Yes?"

"I want you to promise me something."

She looks at me.

"If 400 or Wednesday or any of the others ever tell you that your mommy and daddy don't love you, don't believe them, okay? You know we love you and we always will, right?"

"Yes."

"Have they ever said anything like that?"

"No."

"But if they do, you won't believe them, right?"

"No."

"Good." I nod. "I love you, Jani."

"Love you," she mumbles sleepily.

CHAPTER THIRTY-SIX

June 8, 2009

How many pills did you take?" Ruth, my psychiatrist and the one who prescribes my Lexapro, asks me over the phone. I'm sitting in our car in the bottom of the canyon, the very same one I planned to die in yesterday.

"I don't know exactly. Probably about twenty."

"You are very lucky, Michael. Antidepressants are typically not fatal when one overdoses, but still you are lucky."

"I know."

"Why did you do it?"

Out the window, I see Honey running around, sniffing, and Jani walking around aimlessly, talking to herself.

"I don't really know."

"You are an intelligent man, Michael. You must know why."

"I guess I got tired of fighting." I watch Jani through the window.

She smiles at a person I can't see and claps her hands. "I don't have any hope for the future."

"Why are you are even thinking about the future?"

Her question sounds absurd. "Because my daughter has a disease she'll have for the rest of her life."

"That is true, but you have to go on."

"But I don't know how to do that."

"Michael, nobody knows how to get through life. You do the best you can."

"I've done my best and it wasn't good enough."

"What is it you want, Michael?"

I look at Jani. "I want to help her. I want to take her illness away."

My psychiatrist laughs. "I'm sorry, Michael. You want to cure schizophrenia?" she asks me in her thick Latin accent.

"I just want to make her life easier," I answer, a bit annoyed.

"You are."

This catches me off guard. "How?"

"Never giving up on her."

"I just tried to kill myself, for God's sake."

"You just gave up on yourself."

"I told you. I'm not strong enough."

"Then who is stronger? Tell me. Who is stronger than you? Who could have done a better job?"

"I've made mistakes."

"I would be worried if you hadn't. I would be more worried if you told me you were perfect, but you still haven't answered my question: Who do you think would do a better job than you have?"

"I don't know. Susan, maybe."

"But last year, you told me she was emotionally unable to deal with what was happening to Jani."

"Right now, she's handling it better than I am."

"So the two of you make a pretty good team, then, no?"

I fall silent. She's right. Susan had her moment of weakness and I was there to keep us going. Then, when I broke down, she was there to do the same.

"You each have different weaknesses," my psychiatrist continues, "but together you make one strong person."

I remain silent.

"Okay, here is what I want you to do. No Lexapro for three days. That should be enough time for it to leave your system. Then resume your normal dose."

"Okay."

"And Michael?"

"Yes?"

"Stop trying to be perfect."

I smile. My psychiatrist hangs up.

Jani comes up to the open door and holds out her empty hand. "It's an injured nine," she says, deeply concerned. "It was attacked by a seven. Her leg is broken."

I exhale, cursing myself for telling her that joke: *Why was ten afraid of seven? Because seven eight nine!* Ever since then Jani has talked nonstop about carnivorous numbers. Sevens eat nines. Ones eat eights. Eights eat twos.

Jani looks from her hand to me. "We have to help the nine!"

She expects me to help an invisible number. She's looking to me to "save" one of her hallucinations. What do I do? Tell her she doesn't really have a nine in her hand? That numbers aren't alive and can't be attacked by other numbers?

She looks up at me, her face filled with worry. The number might not be real, but her emotions are.

I get out of the car. "Okay, bring the nine over here."

I go over to the grass beside the road and sit down. I hold out my hands to Jani.

Jani looks at me, confused. "What are you going to do?"

"You want me to help the nine, right? Then you need to give it to me so I can treat it."

Jani puts the hallucination in my hands. "It's a girl nine."

I lower my hands to the grass.

"Don't hurt her!" Jani calls nervously.

"I'm not going to hurt her. First, we need to check her vital signs. How is her breathing?"

Jani kneels on the grass next to me. "Her name is Ninesly."

"You need to focus on your patient, Jani. The first thing you always do is check for the patient's breathing."

"Okay," she answers.

"Is she breathing? If not, we need to start pulmonary resuscitation." Years ago, when I was trying to be a screenwriter, I bought a medical encyclopedia so I could write a spec of a medical show. That, plus the fact that I've spent a lot of time in hospitals lately, has taught me a lot.

Jani leans over the space in the grass between us, putting her hand on Ninesly's invisible chest.

"She's breathing."

"Is the breathing fast, slow, or normal?"

Jani checks. She's completely focused.

"A little bit fast."

"That could be minor hyperventilation due to the stress of the attack. Next, check her heart rate. Is it fast, slow, or normal?"

Jani checks.

"It's also a little fast."

"Okay. Now take Ninesly's blood pressure. If it is low, that could indicate internal bleeding."

Jani pumps an invisible blood pressure cuff. "It's normal."

"Good. That means less likelihood of internal bleeding. Now take her pulse ox."

Jani looks up at me.

"What should it be?"

"In most animals, ninety-five percent and higher is considered normal."

Jani checks. "Ninety-eight."

"That's good. Now you need to take her temperature. A high temperature would indicate a possible infection." I wait while Jani checks the temperature.

"It's normal."

"Okay, we've taken her vital signs. You always do that first before you treat any injuries. You have to make sure your patient is stable."

"What does 'stable' mean?"

"Means she won't die. Now that we've made sure Ninesly is stable, we can treat the leg. She needs to go to Radiology."

Jani gets up and goes over to a tree. "This is Radiology," she announces.

"Do an X-ray of her leg. Is it a single fracture or a compound fracture?"

"Compound."

I breathe out. "Okay, we're going to have to do surgery, then. Start an IV to put her under, plus I need three units of nine blood for Ninesly."

Jani hands me the invisible bags of nine blood.

We go to work, opening Ninesly's leg and inserting pins into the broken bones.

A car drives past. I wonder what the driver thinks. A man and a girl working feverishly over a patch of grass.

I smile. I don't care. Jani is totally focused on the operation to save the leg of her hallucination.

Her world and my world are united.

EPILOGUE

July 2011

The band U2 released their song "Beautiful Day" two years before Jani was born. It's been in heavy rotation ever since. Like Jani's hallucinations, it's still around despite two subsequent albums.

In many ways, "Beautiful Day" represents the duality of my feelings about Jani. In one sense I've both loved and hated this song. Of course, I love the soaring chords, just as I always love Jani. But I hate the chorus and the final refrain.

What you don't have you don't need it now.

When I'd hear the song, I used to say bitterly to Susan, "Easy for Bono to say. He's worth millions. It's easy to tell people they don't need what they don't have when you yourself don't actually need anything." I resented the song, taking it as Bono's celebration of his own glorious life.

By the time Jani went to UCLA, the song had become a slap in my face. *It's a beautiful day* seemed a brutal reminder of how ugly our life had become.

A lot has changed since then. Today, Jani is on three medications: clozapine, lithium, and Thorazine. This combination has been the most successful.

Are her hallucinations completely gone?

No, but as she will tell us, they are not bothering her. It's like having the TV on in the background, volume turned down, while you're doing something, and every so often you look up at the screen to see what 400 the Cat and other hallucinations are doing. They remain on Jani's periphery, but she can still function in our common reality.

Is the violence gone?

Pretty much. By separating Bodhi and Jani into two apartments, we succeeded in what we set out to do, which was to lower Jani's stress level and ensure that Bodhi would not be growing up afraid of his sister. And he isn't. I love hearing the sound of Bodhi's laughter while he and Jani roll around on the floor, playing together.

He calls her his "Si-Si."

We no longer live in constant fear of her hurting him.

The rages are largely gone. I think I've only been hit twice now in the past year.

Is she still antisocial with other kids?

Yes and no. She doesn't play with other kids too often, but in the past year I have seen her walk up to other girls and ask, "What's your name? How old are you?" Every time I see this, it still brings tears to my eyes because there was a time when I thought Jani would never interact with flesh-and-blood people again. It's hard for her because she still sees an entire world they can't, but she no longer seems angry about it. She is trying.

Does she go to school?

Yes. Despite my initial frustrations with our local school district, they're now meeting Jani's needs in a way I never thought possible. She goes to school after all the other kids have left, spending two hours a day receiving education, with periodic breaks as needed, along with additional time spent on occupational therapy, where she often does engage with other special needs kids. She's learning how to type and how to tie her shoelaces. She wants more school but tells us she's not ready to go back into a classroom.

Do we get any help?

Yes, but not from the Department of Mental Health, who to this day *still* wants to send her to an out-of-state residential facility. Actually, the government agency that has helped our family the most has nothing to do with mental illnesses. The help comes from the Los Angeles County Department of Animal Care and Control, specifically the officers and staff at the Castaic, California, Animal Shelter. I started taking Jani there in 2009, and we still go a few times a week. The officers and kennel attendants at the shelter know Jani and let her help take care of the animals. With me by her side, she feeds cats, changes their litter boxes, takes care of the rabbits, reptiles, and even the horses that show up there on occasion. When she was little, she wanted to become a veterinarian, and this hasn't changed. When she's with animals is the only time Jani is completely free of her hallucinations. Beyond Honey, who is thirteen years old now, we have some aquatic turtles (all adopted from the Castaic Animal Shelter) and two betta fish. They are her animal sanctuary and help her focus on something tangible, giving her a common language with which to relate to the rest of the world.

In addition to the shelter, we've gotten help from a place called Carousel Ranch in Agua Dulce, California. They provide equine therapy for physically and mentally disabled kids as well as autistic children. Every week we check in to the office so Jani can take care of "Office Kitty," Carousel Ranch's calico cat. Then it's time for her riding lesson. The wonderful staff teaches her "trick riding." I'm always amazed when I see Jani stand up on the back of the horse and balance on one leg, or ride backward, with the staff supporting her all the way.

While she does this, I muck out the stalls and make sure the horses have water. I do this because Jani gets to ride at Carousel Ranch for free, on a scholarship. I don't have to trade my labor for her lessons, but I want to feel like I'm contributing. I also enjoy it. I find peace in taking care of the horses.

Which brings me back to "Beautiful Day."

There's a twenty-seven-year-old woman, Lucy, who rides at Carousel Ranch at the same time as Jani. Lucy has cerebral palsy, another illness for which there is no cure. She can't just get on the horses like Jani can. She lives most of her life in a wheelchair and has to ride with someone holding her upright, but her smile is always bright and happy when she's up on the horse.

It's a beautiful day, Don't let it get away.

Watching Jani and Lucy ride, I finally get it. The song's not called "Beautiful Life." It's "Beautiful Day," meaning at least this day, today, can be beautiful.

I don't even hope for beautiful days. Every day, in some way, Jani's illness reminds us that it is still there.

But every day there are also moments where I see her smile, moments when I have hope, moments when I feel at peace with our future, whatever might come our way.

These are the moments I live for.

ACKNOWLEDGMENTS

The publication of this book is bittersweet. For obvious reasons, I wish I'd never had to write it. Jani's story is bigger than I am, bigger than any one person, and thankfully there were plenty of people to help me.

I want to thank Stacey Cohen for sharing our story with Shari Roan of the *Los Angeles Times*. I will always be grateful to Shari for seeing the grace in Jani and for refusing to let her become a statistic. My deepest thanks also goes to Erica Wohlreich, Elissa Stohler, and Claire Weinraub, all of whom became part of our family while I was telling Jani's story. Thank you to Oprah, who showed parents all over the world struggling with a mentally ill child that they are not alone.

Thank you to Steve Truitt, who has many titles, but I think "awesome dude" is the best. My attorney, Joshua Binder, and my agent, Byrd Leavell, have gone and continue to go beyond the call of duty in my aid. I hope you both know how lucky I feel to have you as my representatives. If not for you, Byrd, this book never would have been published.

Although they are no longer there, I must thank Christine Pride and Diane Salvatore for their vision of what this story could be and for bringing me to Crown. I deeply thank my wonderful editor, Jenna Ciongoli, for her patience, wisdom, and for her continued faith that I could tell this story even in my darkest hours when I didn't think I could. Thank you so much, Jenna, for hanging in there with me.

Thank you from the bottom of my heart to my friend John Gides. John came the night Jani went into UCLA and I would not have made it without him.

Thank you to my mentor, Jacqueline Mitchard, a far better writer than I will ever be, for challenging me to tell this story.

Thank you to Bethanne, Carl Goss, John Fetto, Dawn, Nancy, Angela, Kelly, Karen, Karlee, Cat, Falcon, Sharone, and all the rest of our "Facebook Family." All of you helped to keep our family going through two difficult years, and I will never forget that. Likewise, thank you to the countless strangers who donated to our family out of the kindness of your hearts.

Thanks to Tony and Anthony. You know why. I owe you a debt I can never repay. A very heartfelt thanks to Jeanne and Lauren for providing Bodhi a safe and happy place during our family's darkest hours.

Thanks to Greg, Ivy, Barry, Jennifer, and Tracy for continuing to be champions for Jani and those like her.

Thanks to Janine Francolini and the Flawless Foundation for turning inspiration into action on behalf of mentally ill kids.

Thank you to Dr. Todd Fine and his wonderful staff of teachers and aides at the Newhall School District. You helped saved Jani's life. The same goes for Dr. W for always fighting to give Jani a better life. Also, my thanks to Dr. DeAntonio and his doctors and nursing staff at the Resnick Neuropsychiatric Hospital. You became Jani's second home and part of her extended family.

A huge thank you to Denise, Becky, Katie, Taylor, and everybody else at Carousel Ranch. You give Jani confidence and hope for the future. I'd say we are a lot better than "fifty/fifty" now.

A huge thank you to Dena, who has become part of our family, as well as Marla Rosenthal for everything she has done.

Thank you to my father for your understanding and never-ending support. By sticking with me during my struggles, you taught me what being a father is about.

Susan. My wife. You helped me so much with this book, your name should be on the cover as well. But more than that, I thank you for sticking by me. I don't know what I did in a previous life to deserve you, but there is no one else I would have wanted by my side.

Thank you to Bodhi for the joy you bring to my life. You may not realize yet what you have done for your sister, but one day you will.

Finally, there is Jani. There are no words in our language to express what I feel for you. You've taken me to places emotionally I never thought I would survive, but seeing you grow despite your illness is the greatest joy of my life. Every day, you challenge me to be a better father and a better human being.

I love you always.

ABOUT THE AUTHOR

M ichael Schofield is a lecturer in English at California State University, Northridge. His family's story has appeared in the *Los Angeles Times* and on *The Oprah Winfrey Show,* ABC's *20/20,* and *Discovery Health.* He lives in the Los Angeles area with his family, now enjoying life together again under one roof. You can follow his family's continuing story as well as contact him at www.janisjourney.org.